Freedom from Obesity

HOW SUCCESSFULLY AND EFFECTIVELY LOSE WEIGHT

MICHAEL FATBURNER

Freedom from Obesity

REAL FANTASY

Michael Fatburner

Real Fantasy

ISBN 978-80-972191-5-4

Editing by Dr. Francis Bartak

Real Fantasy is committed to reducing the consumption
of old-growth forests in the books it publishes. This book is one
step toward that goal.

CONTENTS:

FOREWORD

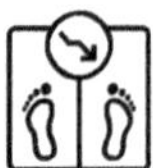

In this book you can find advice from various experts without unnecessary ballast. The publication analyzes tips and strategies from ten personalities in weight loss and healthy lifestyle:

Dr. Katrina Ubell

Author of *How to Lose Weight for the Last Time*, Ubell focuses on brain-based solutions for permanent weight loss, emphasizing emotional awareness and sustainable practices.

Dr. Michael Greger

Founder of NutritionFacts.org and author of *How Not to Die*, Greger advocates for a plant-based diet and provides evidence-based advice on nutrition and weight management.

Dr. Mark Hyman

A functional medicine physician and author of several books, including *Food: What the Heck Should I Eat?*, Hyman emphasizes the role of food in health and weight loss, promoting whole foods and a balanced diet.

Dr. Jason Fung

Known for his work on intermittent fasting and obesity, Fung is the author of *The Obesity Code*, where he discusses the hormonal causes of weight gain and offers strategies for weight loss.

Brooke Castillo

Founder of The Life Coach School, Castillo focuses on the mental aspects of weight loss, teaching clients how to manage their thoughts and emotions around food.

Dr. Phil McGraw

A psychologist and television personality, McGraw has authored several books on weight loss, including *The Ultimate Weight Solution*, which combines psychological principles with practical advice.

Tosca Reno

Author of the *Eat Clean Diet* series, Reno promotes a clean eating lifestyle and has shared her personal weight loss journey through her books and public speaking.

Jillian Michaels

A well-known fitness trainer and television personality, Michaels offers weight loss advice through her books, workout programs, and podcasts, focusing on a combination of diet and exercise.

Dr. James DiNicolantonio

A cardiovascular research scientist and a Doctor of Pharmacy known for his work in nutrition and health. He has written several books, including The Obesity Fix.

Tony Horton

Creator of the P90X fitness program, which combines strength training, cardio, and flexibility workouts to promote weight loss and fitness.

UBELL: HOW TO LOSE WEIGHT FOR THE LAST TIME

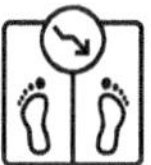

The book *How to Lose Weight for the Last Time* by Dr. Katrina Ubell focuses on brain-based solutions for permanent weight loss, emphasizing the importance of mindset and emotional awareness in the weight loss journey. The main points of Ubells strategy are:

1. **Mindset Shift:** The book stresses changing how we think about food and weight loss, moving away from restrictive diets to a more compassionate and realistic approach.

2. **Understanding Emotions:** Ubell discusses how many people use food to cope with emotions and stresses the need to recognize and address these emotional triggers.

3. **Hunger Awareness:** The concept of the hunger scale is introduced, encouraging readers to listen to their bodies and eat according to genuine hunger rather than external cues or societal pressures.

4. **Sustainable Practices:** The book outlines an 8-point system for maintaining weight loss, focusing on practical tools and strategies that can be easily integrated into daily life.

5. **Avoiding Restrictive Diets:** Ubell advises against cutting out entire food groups, such as sugar and flour, suggesting instead to find a balance that works for the individual.

6. **Behavioral Change:** Emphasis is placed on making lasting changes in thoughts and behaviors around food, rather than relying on temporary diets or exercise regimens.

7. **Personal Experience:** Ubell shares her own struggles with weight and how her experiences have shaped the strategies presented in the book, making it relatable for readers.

Struggles during Weight Loss

Dr. Kathrina Ubell experienced several struggles during her weight loss journey, which she openly discusses in her work and coaching. Here are some key challenges she faced:

1. **Repeated Weight Cycling**

   Dr. Ubell struggled with the cycle of gaining and losing weight multiple times, specifically mentioning that she lost and regained the same 40 pounds at least ten times. This pattern of yo-yo dieting is common among many individuals trying to lose weight, leading to frustration and discouragement when results are not sustained.

2. **Overwhelm and Stress**

   As a busy physician, Dr. Ubell dealt with significant stress and overwhelm, which often led to emotional eating. She recognized that many doctors, including herself, prioritize their patients' needs over their own wellness, making it challenging to focus on personal health and weight management.

3. Lack of Support

Initially, Dr. Ubell felt that as a physician, she should be able to manage her weight without external help. This mindset created a barrier to seeking support and guidance, leading her to believe that struggling with weight loss indicated a personal failure.

4. Misguided Approaches

Dr. Ubell tried numerous diets and weight loss programs, often following methods that emphasized willpower, strict calorie counting, or intense exercise regimens. These approaches were not sustainable for her, as they did not address the underlying psychological and emotional factors contributing to her eating habits.

5. Emotional and Psychological Barriers

She encountered emotional challenges related to body image and self-acceptance, which are common among those attempting to lose weight. Dr. Ubell emphasizes the importance of addressing mental and emotional health in conjunction with physical weight loss efforts.

Conclusion

Through her journey, Dr. Ubell developed a coaching program that focuses on brain-based solutions for permanent weight loss, helping others overcome similar struggles. She emphasizes the need for a compassionate and realistic approach to weight management, integrating personal experiences with scientific insights to support lasting change.

GREGER: HOW NOT TO DIET

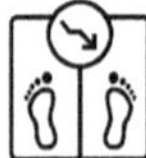

Dr. Michael Greger, a well-known physician and nutrition expert, presents a comprehensive approach to weight loss in his book *How Not to Diet*. His methodology is rooted in scientific research and emphasizes a plant-based diet as a sustainable and effective means to achieve and maintain a healthy weight. Here are the key principles he advocates for successful weight loss:

1. Evidence-Based Approach

Greger's work is distinguished by its reliance on rigorous scientific evidence. He critiques the plethora of anecdotal weight loss stories and focuses instead on what the best available research indicates. His goal is to distill complex scientific findings into practical advice that anyone can follow. He emphasizes that understanding the underlying science of nutrition is crucial for making informed dietary choices.

2. The Ideal Weight-Loss Diet

In *How Not to Diet*, Greger identifies 17 key ingredients that constitute an ideal weight-loss diet. These ingredients are based on their health benefits and their ability to promote weight loss. He stresses that not all calories are equal; for example, 100 calories from chickpeas affect the body differently than 100 calories from processed snacks. This highlights the importance of food quality over mere calorie counting.

3. Focus on Whole, Plant-Based Foods

Greger advocates for a diet rich in whole, plant-based foods, such as fruits, vegetables, whole grains, legumes, nuts, and seeds. These foods are not only low in calories but also high in fiber, which helps to increase satiety and reduce overall calorie intake. He explains that fiber-rich foods can help regulate appetite and improve digestion, making them essential for effective weight management.

4. Understanding Hunger and Satiety

A significant portion of Greger's book is dedicated to understanding the mechanisms of hunger and satiety. He explains how different foods can influence these signals in the body.

For instance, foods high in fiber and water content can help you feel full longer, while processed foods often lead to rapid spikes and crashes in blood sugar, increasing hunger.

5. Timing and Context of Eating

Greger discusses the importance of not just what you eat, but also how and when you eat. He notes that the timing of meals can affect metabolism and fat storage. For example, eating larger meals earlier in the day may be more beneficial than consuming them later. He also emphasizes the impact of meal distribution and the importance of being mindful about when and how much you eat.

6. Behavioral Strategies

In addition to dietary changes, Greger highlights behavioral strategies to support weight loss. He encourages readers to become more aware of their eating habits and emotional triggers that lead to overeating. By recognizing these patterns, individuals can make more conscious choices about their food intake and develop healthier relationships with food.

7. Incorporating Specific Foods and Spices

Greger identifies certain foods and spices that can enhance weight loss efforts. For example, he discusses the benefits of spices like cayenne pepper and cinnamon, which have been shown to boost metabolism and improve fat burning. He encourages readers to incorporate these into their diets to maximize their weight loss potential.

8. Long-Term Sustainability

One of the central themes of Greger's approach is the focus on long-term sustainability rather than quick fixes. He argues that many popular diets are unsustainable and often lead to yo-yo dieting. Instead, he promotes a lifestyle change that can be maintained over time, emphasizing that the goal is not just to lose weight but to achieve overall health and well-being.

Key Ingredients for Ideal Weight-Loss Diet

Dr. Michael Greger identifies 17 key ingredients that constitute an ideal weight-loss diet in his book *How Not to Diet*. These ingredients are based on scientific research and are designed to promote effective and sustainable weight loss. Here's a summary of these ingredients:

1. **Whole Grains**: Foods like brown rice, quinoa, and whole wheat bread are rich in fiber and nutrients, helping to keep you full and satisfied while providing essential energy.

2. **Legumes**: Beans, lentils, and peas are high in protein and fiber, making them excellent for weight management as they promote satiety and have a low glycemic index.

3. **Fruits**: Fresh fruits are packed with vitamins, minerals, and fiber. Their natural sweetness can satisfy cravings for sugary snacks while providing fewer calories.

4. **Vegetables**: Non-starchy vegetables, such as leafy greens, broccoli, and peppers, are low in calories but high in nutrients, making them ideal for filling up without adding excess calories.

5. **Nuts and Seeds**: While calorie-dense, nuts and seeds provide healthy fats, protein, and fiber. They can help curb hunger when consumed in moderation.

6. **Herbs and Spices**: Certain herbs and spices, like cinnamon and cayenne pepper, can enhance flavor without added calories and may even boost metabolism.

7. **Fermented Foods**: Foods like yogurt, kefir, and sauerkraut support gut health, which can influence weight management and overall health.

8. **Healthy Fats**: Sources of healthy fats, such as avocados and olive oil, are essential for nutrient absorption and can help with satiety when consumed in moderation.

9. **Lean Proteins**: Incorporating lean protein sources, such as tofu or skinless poultry, can help maintain muscle mass while losing weight.

10. **Green Tea**: Known for its antioxidant properties, green tea may also aid in weight loss by boosting metabolism and fat oxidation.

11. **Dark Chocolate**: In moderation, dark chocolate can satisfy sweet cravings and provide health benefits due to its antioxidant content.

12. **Potatoes**: Contrary to popular belief, whole potatoes can be part of a healthy diet. They are filling and nutrient-rich when consumed without excessive fats.

13. **Berries**: Berries are low in calories and high in fiber, making them a great option for satisfying sweet cravings while providing antioxidants.

14. **Mushrooms**: Low in calories and high in flavor, mushrooms can be used as a meat substitute in many dishes, helping to reduce overall calorie intake.

15. **Cruciferous Vegetables**: Vegetables like cauliflower and Brussels sprouts are high in fiber and can help with weight loss due to their low calorie density.

16. **Eggs**: When included in moderation, eggs can be a good source of protein and nutrients, helping to keep you full longer.

17. **Fish**: Fatty fish, such as salmon, are rich in omega-3 fatty acids and protein, which can support weight loss and overall health.

Greger emphasizes that the quality of food is more important than merely counting calories. He also discusses how the context in which foods are consumed—such as meal timing and combinations—can significantly impact weight loss success. By focusing on these 17 ingredients, individuals can create a balanced and satisfying diet that supports sustainable weight loss and overall health.

Conclusion

Dr. Michael Greger's *How Not to Diet* offers a science-backed, practical approach to weight loss that prioritizes whole, plant-based foods and sustainable habits. By understanding the science of nutrition and implementing behavioral strategies, individuals can achieve lasting weight loss and improve their overall health. Greger's emphasis on evidence over anecdote provides a refreshing perspective in the often confusing world of dieting, making his guidance valuable for anyone seeking to lose weight effectively and healthily.

HYMAN: THE BLOOD SUGAR SOLUTION

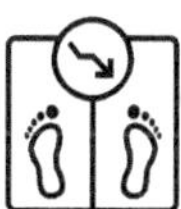

Dr. Mark Hyman, a prominent physician and author, is well-known for his holistic approach to weight loss, particularly through his best-selling book *The Blood Sugar Solution*. His philosophy centers around the connection between diet, metabolism, and overall health, emphasizing that sustainable weight loss is not merely about caloric restriction but involves a comprehensive lifestyle change. Here are the key principles and strategies he advocates for effective weight loss:

1. **Understanding Insulin and Blood Sugar**

   Hyman emphasizes the role of insulin in weight management. He explains that high insulin levels can lead to fat storage, particularly in the abdominal area. To lose weight effectively, it is crucial to maintain low insulin levels.

This can be achieved by reducing the intake of refined carbohydrates and sugars, which cause spikes in blood sugar and insulin. Instead, he promotes a diet that stabilizes blood sugar levels, thereby enhancing fat burning and reducing cravings.

2. The Importance of Whole Foods

Central to Hyman's weight loss strategy is the consumption of whole, unprocessed foods. He advocates for a diet rich in vegetables, fruits, whole grains, lean proteins, and healthy fats. These foods are nutrient-dense and provide the body with essential vitamins and minerals while promoting satiety. Hyman particularly highlights the benefits of plant-based foods, which are lower in calories and high in fiber, aiding in digestion and appetite control.

3. Detoxification

In *The Blood Sugar Solution 10-Day Detox Diet*, Hyman outlines a detoxification process that helps reset the body's metabolism. This involves eliminating processed foods, sugar, and unhealthy fats while introducing detoxifying foods such as leafy greens, cruciferous vegetables, and herbs.

This detox phase is designed to reduce inflammation, improve gut health, and enhance metabolic function, creating a conducive environment for weight loss.

4. Managing Stress and Sleep

Hyman recognizes that stress and inadequate sleep significantly impact weight loss efforts. Chronic stress leads to the release of cortisol, a hormone that can promote fat storage, particularly in the belly area. To combat this, he recommends relaxation techniques such as mindfulness, meditation, and relaxation exercise. Additionally, he stresses the importance of quality sleep, suggesting that individuals aim for 7-9 hours of restful sleep per night to support metabolic health and appetite regulation.

5. Regular Physical Activity

Exercise is another critical component of Hyman's weight loss strategy. He advocates for a balanced approach that includes both aerobic exercises (like walking, running, or cycling) and strength training. Regular physical activity helps to increase metabolism, improve insulin sensitivity, and maintain muscle mass, all of which are essential for effective weight management.

Hyman encourages incorporating movement into daily routines, emphasizing that even small changes can lead to significant health benefits.

6. Behavioral Changes and Mindset

Hyman highlights the importance of addressing the psychological aspects of eating and weight loss. He encourages individuals to become more aware of their eating habits and emotional triggers that lead to overeating. Journaling and mindfulness practices can help individuals identify patterns and develop healthier relationships with food. By fostering a positive mindset and focusing on long-term health rather than short-term results, individuals are more likely to sustain their weight loss efforts.

7. Personalization of Diet Plans

Recognizing that there is no one-size-fits-all approach to weight loss, Hyman emphasizes the need for personalized dietary strategies. He encourages individuals to listen to their bodies and adjust their diets based on their unique needs, preferences, and health conditions. This may include experimenting with different macronutrient ratios or meal timing to find what works best for them.

8. Incorporating Supplements Wisely

While Hyman advocates for obtaining nutrients primarily through whole foods, he acknowledges that certain supplements can support weight loss and overall health. For example, omega-3 fatty acids, vitamin D, and probiotics may help improve metabolic function and gut health. However, he stresses that supplements should complement a healthy diet, not replace it.

9. Avoiding Processed Foods and Sugars

Hyman strongly advises against the consumption of processed foods and added sugars. These foods not only contribute to weight gain but also lead to inflammation and various health issues. He encourages individuals to read labels carefully and choose foods with minimal ingredients, focusing on those that are whole and natural.

10. Creating a Supportive Environment

Lastly, Hyman emphasizes the importance of a supportive environment for successful weight loss. This includes surrounding oneself with like-minded individuals who encourage healthy habits, as well as making changes in the home environment to reduce temptations.

Meal planning and preparation can also play a significant role in staying on track with dietary goals.

10-Day Detox Diet

The key of 10-Day Detox Diet is to make sustainable changes that support your body's natural detoxification processes. By focusing on whole foods, reducing toxins, managing stress, and incorporating healthy lifestyle habits, you can experience improved energy, weight loss, and overall well-being.

Preparation Phase

- Clean out your pantry and fridge, removing processed foods, sugary drinks, and unhealthy items

- Stock up on whole foods like vegetables, fruits, lean proteins, nuts, and healthy fats

- Set your intentions and align your mindset for success

- Join a supportive community to double your results

Diet Plan

- Eat a diet focused on whole, unprocessed foods

  - Vegetables (especially leafy greens, cruciferous veggies, artichokes, asparagus)

  - Fruits (berries, citrus fruits, apples)

  - Lean proteins (grass-fed beef, poultry, salmon, tuna)

  - Healthy fats (avocados, olive oil, nuts and seeds)

  - Whole grains (in moderation)

- Drink plenty of water (at least 8 glasses per day)

- Limit or eliminate alcohol and caffeine

- Exercise regularly (aim for 30 minutes of moderate activity daily)

- Get 7-8 hours of quality sleep each night

- Practice relaxation techniques like meditation, deep breathing, and relaxation exercise

- Take recommended supplements to support detoxification

- Track your progress, measurements, and experiences in a journal

Transition Phase

- Gradually reintroduce foods while maintaining healthy habits

- Identify trigger foods and develop a long-term plan for sustained health

Conclusion

Dr. Mark Hyman's approach to weight loss is comprehensive, focusing on the interplay between diet, lifestyle, and overall health. By understanding the role of insulin, prioritizing whole foods, managing stress, and fostering a positive mindset, individuals can achieve sustainable weight loss and improve their overall well-being. Hyman's strategies are designed not just for quick fixes but for long-term health, making them applicable to anyone seeking to lose weight effectively and maintain a healthy lifestyle.

FUNG: THE OBESITY CODE

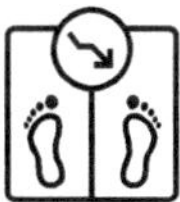

Dr. Jason Fung, a prominent nephrologist and author, has gained recognition for his work on intermittent fasting and its role in weight loss and metabolic health. In his book *The Obesity Code*, Fung presents a comprehensive approach to understanding and addressing the root causes of obesity. Here are the key principles he advocates for effective and sustainable weight loss:

1. **Understanding Insulin and Insulin Resistance**

   Central to Fung's approach is the concept of insulin resistance, which he believes is the primary driver of obesity. He explains that high insulin levels, often caused by a diet high in refined carbohydrates and sugars, can lead to fat storage and difficulty losing weight. By reducing insulin levels through dietary changes and intermittent fasting, the body can more effectively burn fat for fuel.

2. The Role of Intermittent Fasting

Fung emphasizes the importance of intermittent fasting in his weight loss strategy. He suggests that by cycling between periods of eating and fasting, the body can reset its sensitivity to insulin and optimize fat burning. Fung recommends various fasting protocols, such as the 16/8 method (fasting for 16 hours and eating within an 8-hour window) or the 24-hour fast (fasting for a full day once or twice a week). He stresses that the key is to find a fasting regimen that works best for the individual and their lifestyle.

3. Macronutrient Balance

While Fung acknowledges that calorie restriction can lead to weight loss, he argues that the quality of the calories is more important than the quantity. He suggests focusing on a diet that is low in refined carbohydrates and high in healthy fats and proteins. This macronutrient balance helps to stabilize blood sugar levels and reduce insulin resistance, making it easier to lose weight and maintain a healthy metabolism.

4. Addressing Hormonal Imbalances

Fung recognizes that hormonal imbalances, such as thyroid dysfunction or polycystic ovary syndrome (PCOS), can contribute to weight gain and make it challenging to lose weight. He recommends working with a healthcare professional to identify and address any underlying hormonal issues that may be hindering weight loss efforts.

5. Stress Management and Sleep

Fung emphasizes the importance of managing stress and getting adequate sleep in his weight loss approach. Chronic stress can lead to the release of cortisol, a hormone that can promote fat storage and disrupt metabolism. He suggests incorporating stress-reducing activities into daily routines. Additionally, Fung stresses the importance of prioritizing sleep, as sleep deprivation has been linked to increased hunger, decreased satiety, and impaired insulin sensitivity.

6. Individualized Approach

Fung acknowledges that there is no one-size-fits-all solution to weight loss. He encourages individuals to experiment with different fasting protocols and dietary approaches to find what works best for their unique body and lifestyle. He emphasizes the importance of listening to one's body and making adjustments as needed to achieve optimal results.

7. Sustainability and Mindset

Fung emphasizes the importance of sustainability and mindset in his weight loss approach. He encourages individuals to view weight loss as a long-term lifestyle change rather than a temporary fix. By adopting a positive mindset and focusing on the health benefits of weight loss, individuals are more likely to stick to their goals and maintain their results over time.

Low Refined Carbohydrates

Dr. Jason Fung advocates for a diet that is low in refined carbohydrates and high in healthy fats and proteins to support weight loss and metabolic health. Here are examples of foods that fit this dietary approach:

1. **Whole Grains**:

    - **Quinoa**: A nutrient-rich grain that is high in protein and fiber.

    - **Brown Rice**: A whole grain that provides more fiber and nutrients than white rice.

    - **Oats**: Particularly steel-cut or rolled oats, which are high in fiber and help regulate blood sugar levels.

2. **Non-Starchy Vegetables**:

    - **Leafy Greens**: Spinach, kale, and Swiss chard are low in calories and high in nutrients.

- **Cruciferous Vegetables**: Broccoli, cauliflower, and Brussels sprouts are excellent choices that are low in carbohydrates.

- **Bell Peppers**: Rich in vitamins and low in calories, they add flavor and nutrition to meals.

3. **Legumes**:

   - **Lentils**: High in protein and fiber, they help keep you full and satisfied.

   - **Chickpeas**: Versatile and nutritious, they can be used in salads, stews, or made into hummus.

   - **Black Beans**: A great source of protein and fiber, they can be added to various dishes.

4. **Healthy Fats**

   - **Avocados**: Packed with monounsaturated fats, avocados are nutritious and help increase satiety.

   - **Almonds**: High in healthy fats and protein, they make for a great snack.

- **Chia Seeds**: Rich in omega-3 fatty acids and fiber, they can be added to smoothies, yogurt, or oatmeal.

- **Walnuts**: Another source of healthy fats, walnuts also provide protein and fiber.

- **Olive Oil**: A staple of the Mediterranean diet, extra virgin olive oil is high in monounsaturated fats and antioxidants.

- **Coconut Oil**: Contains medium-chain triglycerides (MCTs), which may help with weight loss and metabolic health.

5. High-Quality Proteins

- **Salmon**: Rich in omega-3 fatty acids and protein, salmon is beneficial for heart health and satiety.

- **Sardines**: Packed with nutrients and healthy fats, they can be a convenient source of protein.

- **Shellfish**: Such as shrimp and crab, are low in calories and high in protein.

- **Chicken Breast**: A lean source of protein that can be prepared in various ways.

- **Turkey**: Another lean protein option that is versatile for cooking.

- **Eggs:** Whole eggs are nutrient-dense and high in protein. They can help increase feelings of fullness.

- **Tofu and Tempeh**: Excellent sources of protein for vegetarians and vegans, they can be used in a variety of dishes.

- **Edamame**: Young soybeans that are high in protein and fiber.

- **Greek Yogurt**: High in protein and probiotics, Greek yogurt can be a healthy snack or breakfast option.

- **Cottage Cheese**: A low-fat, high-protein dairy option that can be eaten on its own or added to meals.

Conclusion

Dr. Jason Fung's approach to weight loss is centered around the principles of insulin regulation, intermittent fasting, and a focus on overall metabolic health.

By understanding the role of insulin in fat storage and utilizing fasting protocols, individuals can effectively lose weight and improve their metabolic markers. Fung's emphasis on individualization, stress management, and sustainability sets his approach apart, making it a viable option for those seeking a comprehensive and evidence-based weight loss strategy.

Dr. Jason Fung's dietary recommendations focus on whole, unprocessed foods that are low in refined carbohydrates and high in healthy fats and proteins. This approach not only supports weight loss but also promotes overall health and metabolic function. By incorporating foods such as whole grains, non-starchy vegetables, legumes, healthy fats, and high-quality proteins, individuals can create a balanced and satisfying diet that aids in weight management and improves overall well-being.

CASTILLO: PSYCHOLOGICAL FACTORS THAT DRIVE OUR BEHAVIORS

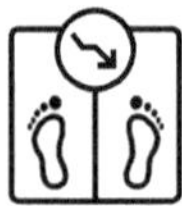

Brooke Castillo, a prominent life coach and weight loss expert, offers a unique approach to weight loss that focuses on the emotional and cognitive aspects of overeating. In her work, Castillo emphasizes that weight loss is not just about restricting calories or following a specific diet, but rather about addressing the underlying emotional and psychological factors that drive our eating behaviors.

1. **Understanding the Root Causes of Overeating**

   Castillo believes that overeating is often a symptom of deeper emotional issues that we are trying to avoid or cope with. She explains that the reasons why we overeat have nothing to do with food itself, but rather with what's going on in our minds and emotions.

By becoming more aware of our thoughts and feelings, we can start to address the root causes of our overeating behaviors.

2. Developing Self-Awareness and Self-Compassion

One of the key principles in Castillo's approach is the importance of developing self-awareness and self compassion. She emphasizes that in order to make lasting changes, we need to be willing to look at ourselves honestly and with kindness. This means acknowledging our struggles and challenges without irrational judgment, and treating ourselves with the same compassion we would extend to a friend.

3. Changing Our Thoughts and Beliefs

Castillo's method also involves changing our thoughts and beliefs about food, our bodies, and ourselves. She believes that many of our struggles with weight are rooted in negative thought patterns and limiting beliefs that we have internalized over time.

By becoming aware of these thoughts and challenging them with more empowering beliefs, we can start to break free from the cycle of overeating and self-criticism.

4. Embracing Discomfort and Uncertainty

Another important aspect of Castillo's approach is the idea of embracing discomfort and uncertainty. She acknowledges that making changes to our eating habits and relationship with food can be challenging and uncomfortable at times. However, she encourages her clients to lean into these feelings, knowing that they are a necessary part of the growth process. By learning to tolerate discomfort and sit with uncertainty, we can build resilience and develop the skills we need to navigate life's ups and downs without turning to food for comfort.

5. Focusing on Progress Over Perfection

Castillo also emphasizes the importance of focusing on progress over perfection when it comes to weight loss. She recognizes that there will be setbacks and challenges along the way, but encourages her clients to celebrate small wins and keep moving forward.

By letting go of the idea of perfection and embracing a growth mindset, we can learn from our mistakes and continue to make progress towards our goals.

6. Prioritizing Self-Care and Balance

Finally, Castillo emphasizes the importance of prioritizing self-care and balance in our lives. She believes that true and lasting weight loss requires a holistic approach that addresses all aspects of our well-being, including our physical, emotional, and mental health. By making time for activities that nourish and support us, such as exercise, meditation, and spending time with loved ones, we can create a foundation for sustainable change.

Conclusion

Brooke Castillo's approach to weight loss is a refreshing departure from traditional dieting methods that focus solely on calorie restriction and macronutrient ratios. By addressing the emotional and psychological aspects of overeating, Castillo helps her clients develop a healthier and more sustainable relationship with food and their bodies.

Through her emphasis on self-awareness, self-compassion, and embracing discomfort, she empowers her clients to make lasting changes that go beyond just the number on the scale. Ultimately, Castillo's approach is about more than just losing weight - it's about reclaiming our power, embracing our true selves, and living a life that feels authentic and fulfilling.

McGRAW: THE 7 KEYS TO WEIGHT LOSS FREEDOM

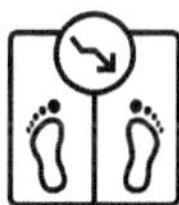

Dr. Phil McGraw, a well-known psychologist and television personality, has developed a comprehensive approach to weight loss that emphasizes the importance of changing not just what you eat, but also how you think about food and your relationship with it. His philosophy is encapsulated in his book, *The Ultimate Weight Solution: The 7 Keys to Weight Loss Freedom*, where he outlines a holistic strategy for achieving and maintaining a healthy weight.

1. The Importance of Lifestyle Change

Dr. Phil asserts that to lose weight and keep it off, individuals must undergo significant lifestyle changes. This includes altering their eating habits, exercise routines, and even their social environments.

He emphasizes that quick-fix diets are generally ineffective in the long term, as they do not address the underlying behaviors and thought patterns that contribute to weight gain. Instead, he advocates for a sustainable approach that involves making gradual changes to one's lifestyle.

2. The Seven Keys to Weight Loss Freedom

In his book, Dr. Phil outlines seven key components that he believes are essential for successful weight loss:

- **Key 1: The Right Mindset**

  McGraw emphasizes the necessity of a positive mindset. He suggests that individuals need to believe in their ability to lose weight and maintain that loss. This involves setting realistic goals and developing a strong motivation to change.

- **Key 2: The Power of Choice**

  Dr. Phil stresses that individuals have the power to make choices about what they eat and how they live. He encourages readers to take responsibility for their decisions and to consciously choose healthier options.

- **Key 3: The Importance of a Support System**

  Having a supportive network of friends and family can significantly impact weight loss success. Dr. Phil recommends surrounding oneself with positive influences that encourage healthy behaviors.

- **Key 4: The Role of Nutrition**

  Nutrition is a cornerstone of Dr. Phil's approach. He advises focusing on whole, nutrient-dense foods while minimizing processed foods and sugars. He introduces the concept of "high-response cost foods," which require more effort to prepare and eat, helping to prevent overeating.

- **Key 5: The Need for Exercise**

  Regular physical activity is crucial for weight loss and overall health. Dr. Phil encourages incorporating exercise into daily routines, emphasizing that it doesn't have to be overly strenuous. Finding enjoyable activities can make exercise more sustainable.

- **Key 6: The Management of Emotions**

  Emotional eating is a significant barrier to weight loss for many individuals. Dr. Phil encourages readers to identify their emotional triggers and develop healthier coping mechanisms. This may involve journaling, therapy, or other strategies to manage stress and emotions without turning to food.

- **Key 7: The Importance of Accountability**

  Accountability plays a vital role in the weight loss journey. Dr. Phil suggests tracking progress, whether through a food diary, regular weigh-ins, or support groups. This accountability helps individuals stay committed to their goals.

3. The 20/20 Diet

In addition to his original weight loss principles, Dr. Phil has introduced the *20/20 Diet*, which focuses on a structured eating plan. This diet consists of four phases:

- **Phase 1: The Five-Day Boost**

  This initial phase involves consuming a limited selection of 20 specific foods designed to kickstart weight loss and help individuals detox from unhealthy eating habits.

- **Phase 2: The Five-Day Sustain**

  In this phase, more foods are gradually reintroduced, but meals must still include at least two of the original 20 foods. This helps maintain the momentum of weight loss while allowing for more variety.

- **Phase 3: The 20-Day Sustain**

  This phase allows for even more food options, with the goal of establishing a sustainable eating pattern. Individuals are encouraged to eat four meals spaced four hours apart, with two splurges allowed each week.

- **Phase 4: The Management Phase**

  This final phase focuses on maintaining weight loss through continued healthy eating habits and lifestyle changes. Dr. Phil emphasizes the importance of ongoing commitment to prevent regaining weight.

4. The Role of Cognitive Behavioral Techniques

Dr. Phil integrates cognitive behavioral techniques into his weight loss approach, helping individuals reframe their thoughts about food and their bodies. He encourages readers to challenge negative beliefs and replace them with positive affirmations. This mental shift is crucial for developing a healthier relationship with food and fostering long-term success.

The 20/20 Diet – Five-Day-Boost Phase

The 20/20 Diet developed by Dr. Phil McGraw consists of a "five-day boost" phase where you kickstart the weight loss process by only eating 20 specific power foods. These 20 foods are:

- coconut oil

- green tea

- mustard

- olive oil

- almonds

- apples

- chickpeas

- dried plums

- prunes

- leafy greens

- lentils

- peanut butter

- pistachios

- raisins

- yogurt

- eggs

- cod

- rye

- tofu

- whey powder

The 20/20 Diet aims to eat these 20 foods that take a lot of energy to break down, which may increase calorie burn rate and keep you full. This limited selection of foods is used only in the initial five-day boost phase to kickstart weight loss before gradually reintroducing more foods in the later phases of the diet.

The 20/20 Diet – Next Phases

In the later phases of Dr. Phil McGraw's 20/20 Diet, participants are allowed to reintroduce a wider variety of foods beyond the initial 20 power foods. Here's a breakdown of the foods that can be included in each of the subsequent phases:

Phase 2: The 5-Day Sustain

During this phase, which follows the initial five-day boost, individuals can introduce additional foods while still incorporating at least two of the original 20 power foods in every meal and snack. Recommended foods to add include:

- **Fruits**: Blueberries, strawberries, and other berries.

- **Vegetables**: Carrots, tomatoes, and mushrooms.

- **Grains**: Oats and brown rice.

- **Protein**: Chicken breast and tuna.

- **Nuts**: Cashews.

This phase allows for a bit more flexibility while maintaining the core principles of the diet.

Phase 3: The 20-Day Attain

In this phase, participants can further expand their food choices while still adhering to the diet's structure. Foods that can be introduced include:

- **Fruits**: Avocados, raspberries, and bananas.

- **Vegetables**: Potatoes and spinach.

- **Grains**: Quinoa and other whole grains.

- **Legumes**: Black beans and lentils.

- **Healthy Fats**: Additional nuts and seeds.

During this 20-day phase, individuals are encouraged to continue eating at least one of the original power foods in each meal and can also enjoy two "sensible splurges" per week, which are treats kept under 100 calories each.

Phase 4: Management

After reaching their weight loss goals, participants enter the management phase, where they maintain the healthy eating habits established in the previous phases. The focus is on sustaining weight loss through:

- Continuing to incorporate a variety of fruits and vegetables.

- Eating lean proteins like chicken, turkey, and fish.

- Including healthy fats like avocados, nuts, and olive oil.

- Monitoring portion sizes and maintaining regular meal timing.

In this phase, individuals are encouraged to develop a balanced lifestyle that includes regular exercise, hydration, and mindful eating practices to prevent weight regain.

Summary

The 20/20 Diet progresses from a strict regimen of 20 power foods to a more flexible approach that allows for a variety of nutritious options. In the later phases, participants can introduce fruits, vegetables, whole grains, lean proteins, and healthy fats, all while maintaining the foundational principles of the diet. This structured yet adaptable approach aims to promote sustainable weight loss and a healthier relationship with food.

Conclusion

Dr. Phil McGraw's approach to weight loss is comprehensive and multifaceted, focusing on the interplay between mindset, nutrition, exercise, and emotional well-being. By emphasizing the importance of lifestyle changes and providing practical strategies through his seven keys and the *20/20 Diet*, he empowers individuals to take control of their weight loss journey.

His philosophy encourages a holistic view of health, recognizing that true weight loss success involves not just changes in diet, but also in how we think, feel, and interact with food. By addressing the psychological aspects of eating and fostering a supportive environment, Dr. Phil aims to help individuals achieve lasting weight loss and improved overall health.

RENO: THE EAT CLEAN DIET

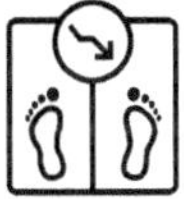

Tosca Reno, a renowned nutrition expert and author of the Eat-Clean Diet series, has developed a comprehensive approach to weight loss that emphasizes the importance of clean eating, balanced nutrition, and lifestyle changes. Her philosophy revolves around the idea that food can be both nourishing and enjoyable, and that sustainable weight loss is achievable through mindful eating and healthy habits. Here's a detailed look at her strategies for effective weight loss.

1. The Philosophy of Clean Eating

At the core of Tosca Reno's approach is the concept of clean eating, which involves consuming whole, unprocessed foods while avoiding artificial ingredients, preservatives, and refined sugars.

Reno defines clean eating as choosing foods that are as close to their natural state as possible.

This means prioritizing fresh fruits, vegetables, whole grains, lean proteins, and healthy fats. By focusing on nutrient-dense foods, individuals can improve their overall health and facilitate weight loss without the need for restrictive diets.

2. Meal Frequency and Portion Control

Reno advocates for eating smaller, more frequent meals throughout the day, typically five to six meals. This approach helps to maintain stable blood sugar levels, control hunger, and prevent overeating. Each meal should include a balance of lean protein, complex carbohydrates, and healthy fats. Reno emphasizes the importance of portion control, encouraging individuals to listen to their bodies and eat until they are satisfied, not stuffed.

3. The Role of Sugar Detox

One of Reno's signature programs is the Strike Sugar plan, which focuses on detoxifying the body from sugar and reducing cravings. She believes that sugar is a significant contributor to weight gain and unhealthy eating habits. The sugar detox involves eliminating refined sugars and processed foods from the diet, which can help individuals regain control over their cravings and improve their overall health. Reno suggests replacing sugary snacks with healthier alternatives, such as fruits, nuts, and yogurt, to satisfy sweet cravings without the negative effects of sugar.

4. Emphasizing Nutrient-Dense Foods

Reno encourages individuals to incorporate a variety of nutrient-dense foods into their diets. This includes:

Lean Proteins: Sources such as chicken, turkey, fish, tofu, and legumes help build muscle and keep you full.

Whole Grains: Foods like quinoa, brown rice, and whole wheat bread provide essential fiber and energy.

Healthy Fats: Incorporating sources like avocados, nuts, seeds, and olive oil supports overall health and satiety.

Fruits and Vegetables: A wide variety of colorful fruits and vegetables ensures a rich intake of vitamins, minerals, and antioxidants.

By focusing on these nutrient-dense foods, individuals can create meals that are satisfying and supportive of their weight loss goals.

5. Mindful Eating Practices

Reno emphasizes the importance of mindfulness in eating. This involves being present during meals, savoring each bite, and paying attention to hunger and fullness cues. Mindful eating helps individuals develop a healthier relationship with food, reducing emotional eating and mindless snacking. Reno encourages practices such as eating without distractions, appreciating the flavors and textures of food, and taking the time to enjoy meals.

6. Regular Physical Activity

In addition to dietary changes, Reno advocates for regular physical activity as a crucial component of weight loss.

She recommends incorporating both cardiovascular exercise and strength training into a weekly routine. Activities such as walking, running, cycling, and weightlifting help burn calories, build muscle, and improve overall fitness. Reno suggests finding enjoyable activities to make exercise a sustainable part of one's lifestyle.

7. Emotional Self-Care

Reno recognizes that emotional well-being plays a significant role in weight management. She encourages individuals to address emotional eating by identifying triggers and developing healthier coping mechanisms. This may involve journaling, seeking support from friends or professionals, and practicing stress-reduction techniques such as meditation. By focusing on emotional self-care, individuals can create a more balanced approach to weight loss.

8. Building a Supportive Environment

Creating a supportive environment is essential for successful weight loss. Reno advises surrounding oneself with positive influences, whether through friends, family, or support groups. Having a network of people who encourage healthy habits can make a significant difference in motivation and accountability. Additionally,

Reno suggests decluttering the kitchen of unhealthy foods and stocking it with clean eating options to make healthier choices easier.

9. Long-Term Sustainability

Reno emphasizes that weight loss should not be viewed as a temporary fix but as a long-term lifestyle change. She encourages individuals to set realistic goals and be patient with themselves throughout the process. By focusing on gradual changes and celebrating small victories, individuals can create lasting habits that support their health and well-being.

Eat Smaller, More Frequent

Tosca Reno's approach to eating smaller, more frequent meals throughout the day is a key component of her *Eat-Clean Diet* strategy for weight loss and overall health. Here's a more detailed look at this specific aspect of her philosophy:

The Benefits of Eating Smaller, More Frequent Meals

Reno advocates for consuming five to six meals per day, spaced evenly throughout the day. This approach offers several benefits:

1. **Maintaining Blood Sugar Levels**: Eating smaller meals helps keep blood sugar levels stable, preventing spikes and crashes that can lead to cravings and overeating.

2. **Controlling Hunger**: Frequent meals help manage hunger and prevent extreme feelings of hunger, which can make it easier to make healthy choices.

3. **Boosting Metabolism**: While the effect is modest, eating more frequently may slightly increase metabolism by requiring the body to expend energy digesting food more often.

4. **Portion Control**: Smaller meals make it easier to control portions and avoid overeating at any given time.

Meal Composition

Each of the five to six meals should include a balance of lean protein, complex carbohydrates, and healthy fats.

This combination helps keep you feeling full and satisfied while providing sustained energy. Reno suggests:

- **Lean Proteins**: Chicken, turkey, fish, tofu, legumes, and eggs

- **Complex Carbohydrates**: Whole grains like quinoa, brown rice, and whole wheat bread

- **Healthy Fats**: Avocados, nuts, seeds, and olive oil

Reno emphasizes the importance of choosing nutrient-dense, whole food sources for each macronutrient to maximize the nutritional value of each meal.

Meal Planning and Preparation

To make eating smaller, more frequent meals feasible, Reno recommends planning and preparing meals in advance. This may involve:

- **Batch Cooking**: Preparing larger portions of lean proteins, whole grains, and roasted vegetables to use throughout the week

- **Packing Snacks**: Having healthy snacks like fresh fruit, raw veggies, and nuts readily available to eat between meals

- **Keeping a Food Journal**: Tracking meals and snacks to ensure consistency with the five to six meal plan

Planning ahead helps eliminate the need to make rushed decisions that may lead to unhealthy choices.

Adjusting to the Frequent Meal Schedule

Reno acknowledges that transitioning to eating five to six meals per day may take some time and adjustment. She suggests:

- **Starting Gradually**: Begin with three to four meals per day and gradually increase to five to six over time

- **Listening to Your Body**: Pay attention to hunger and fullness cues to determine the optimal meal frequency for your individual needs

- **Staying Hydrated**: Drink plenty of water throughout the day to support digestion and prevent mistaking thirst for hunger

With practice and consistency, eating smaller, more frequent meals can become a sustainable habit that supports weight loss and overall health.

Conclusion

Tosca Reno's approach to weight loss is rooted in the principles of clean eating, mindful practices, and holistic well-being. By focusing on whole, nutrient-dense foods, regular physical activity, and emotional self-care, individuals can achieve sustainable weight loss and improve their overall health. Reno's philosophy encourages a positive relationship with food and promotes a lifestyle that is both enjoyable and fulfilling. Through her programs and guidance, she empowers individuals to take control of their health and make lasting changes that enhance their quality of life.

Tosca Reno's strategy of eating five to six smaller meals throughout the day is designed to help individuals maintain stable blood sugar levels, control hunger, and make healthier choices.

By planning ahead and choosing nutrient-dense whole foods, this approach can be an effective tool for weight loss and long-term wellness. As with any dietary change, it's essential to listen to your body and adjust the plan as needed to find what works best for you.

MICHAELS: THE BIGGEST LOSER

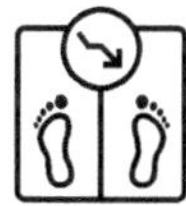

Jillian Michaels, a well-known fitness expert and former trainer on NBC's *The Biggest Loser*, has developed a comprehensive approach to weight loss that combines effective exercise, balanced nutrition, and psychological strategies. Over her extensive career, she has shared numerous insights on how to achieve sustainable weight loss. Here's an overview of her key principles and strategies for losing weight effectively.

1. Focus on Balanced Nutrition

Michaels emphasizes the importance of a balanced diet that includes all three macronutrients: carbohydrates, proteins, and fats. She advocates for whole, nutrient-dense foods while minimizing processed foods and added sugars. Her approach encourages individuals to ask themselves three questions at every meal:

- **Where's my protein?**

- **Where's my fiber?**

- **Where's my healthy fat?**

By ensuring that each meal contains these elements, individuals can promote satiety and maintain energy levels throughout the day. Lean proteins, such as chicken, turkey, fish, and plant-based options like beans and tofu, are emphasized for their role in muscle maintenance and recovery.

2. Avoid Fad Diets

Michaels strongly advises against following fad diets that promise quick results but are often unsustainable. She warns that extreme diets can harm metabolism and lead to yo-yo dieting. Instead, she encourages a common-sense approach to eating, which involves making healthier choices without feeling deprived. This includes understanding portion sizes and listening to one's body to avoid overeating.

3. Hydration is Key

Michaels highlights the importance of hydration in weight loss. Drinking water can help curb hunger and boost metabolism. She recommends drinking water throughout the day and suggests that individuals should aim for hydration levels that keep their urine light yellow, indicating proper hydration. Additionally, she emphasizes that drinking calories, such as sugary beverages, should be avoided to prevent unnecessary calorie intake.

4. Incorporate Regular Exercise

Physical activity is a cornerstone of Michaels' weight loss philosophy. She advocates for a combination of high-intensity interval training (HIIT) and resistance training, as these methods are effective for burning calories and building muscle. HIIT workouts are particularly beneficial because they can be completed in a shorter amount of time while still providing significant calorie-burning benefits.Michaels encourages individuals to find exercises they enjoy, as this increases the likelihood of consistency. Whether it's dancing, running, or strength training, enjoying the workout is crucial for long-term adherence. She also recommends changing up workout routines regularly to prevent plateaus and keep things interesting.

5. Mindset and Motivation

Michaels believes that mindset plays a vital role in weight loss success. She encourages individuals to focus on health rather than just aesthetics. By shifting the focus from body image to overall well-being, individuals may find it easier to stay motivated and committed to their goals. She also emphasizes the importance of setting realistic and achievable goals, celebrating small victories along the way, and maintaining a positive attitude.

6. Address Emotional Eating

Understanding and addressing emotional eating is another critical aspect of Michaels' approach. She suggests that individuals identify their emotional triggers and find healthier coping mechanisms. This may involve journaling, seeking support from friends or professionals, or practicing mindfulness techniques. By recognizing the emotional aspects of eating, individuals can develop a healthier relationship with food.

7. Smart Snacking

Michaels advocates for smart snacking as a strategy to prevent overeating at main meals.

She recommends preparing healthy snacks in advance, such as fruits, vegetables, nuts, or yogurt, to have on hand when hunger strikes. This helps to keep energy levels stable and prevents the temptation to reach for unhealthy options.

8. Rest and Recovery

Michaels emphasizes the importance of rest and recovery in a weight loss program. She recommends incorporating rest days into workout routines to allow the body to recover and prevent injury. Additionally, adequate sleep is crucial for weight management, as lack of sleep can lead to increased hunger and cravings. She suggests aiming for 7-9 hours of quality sleep each night.

9. Use Technology to Your Advantage

Michaels encourages the use of fitness apps and technology to track progress and stay accountable. Her own app provides personalized workout plans, meal suggestions, and tracking tools to help users stay on track with their fitness goals. By utilizing technology, individuals can easily monitor their progress and make adjustments as needed.

10. Stay Consistent

Finally, Michaels stresses the importance of consistency in achieving weight loss goals. She believes that sustainable weight loss is a journey that requires commitment and perseverance. By making small, manageable changes to one's lifestyle and sticking with them, individuals can achieve lasting results.

Portion Sizes as a Key Strategy

Jillian Michaels emphasizes the importance of understanding portion sizes as a key strategy for weight loss and maintenance. Here are some of the ways she approaches portion control:

Avoid Overeating, Even with Healthy Foods

Michaels stresses that weight loss and maintenance are ultimately about the quantity of food consumed, not just the quality. Even if you're eating healthy foods like hummus, kale, chicken, and oatmeal, overeating can still prevent weight loss. She advises, "Don't overeat! Granted, healthier foods will do a better job of fueling your body, but at the end of the day, a calorie is a calorie."

Use Visual Cues for Portion Sizes

To help gauge appropriate portion sizes, Michaels suggests using visual references:

- A palm-sized portion for protein

- A fist-sized portion for complex carbs

- A thumb-sized portion for healthy fats

- Unlimited amounts of non-starchy vegetables

This makes it easier to eyeball proper portions without having to measure everything.

Plate Your Food Strategically

Michaels recommends using a smaller plate to control portions. Filling a 9-inch plate with 50% non-starchy veggies, 25% lean protein, and 25% complex carbs can help ensure you get a balanced meal with appropriate portions.

Slow Down and Savor Your Food

Eating too quickly can lead to overeating, as it takes time for your brain to register feelings of fullness.

Michaels advises slowing down and savoring each bite to allow your body to recognize when you've had enough. Put your fork down between bites and focus on the flavors and textures of your food.

Avoid Eating Straight from Containers

Eating directly from bags, boxes or containers makes it easy to overeat without realizing it. Michaels suggests portioning out a single serving onto a plate or bowl before eating to be more mindful of how much you're consuming.

Drink Water Before Meals

Drinking a glass of water before a meal can help fill you up and prevent overeating. Michaels notes that thirst is often mistaken for hunger, so staying hydrated throughout the day is important.

Manage Portions When Eating Out

Restaurants often serve oversized portions. Michaels suggests splitting an entree with a friend, ordering an appetizer as a main dish, or asking for a to-go box at the start of the meal to portion out half to take home.

By implementing these portion control strategies, Michaels believes individuals can lose weight and maintain their results in a healthy, sustainable way. The key is to be mindful of how much you're eating, even of nutritious foods, and to make adjustments to portions as needed based on your individual goals and needs.

Conclusion

Jillian Michaels' approach to weight loss is comprehensive and multifaceted, focusing on balanced nutrition, regular exercise, mindset, and emotional well-being. By emphasizing the importance of whole foods, hydration, and a positive mindset, she empowers individuals to take control of their health and make sustainable changes. Her philosophy encourages a holistic view of weight loss, recognizing that true success involves not just losing weight, but also improving overall health and well-being. Through her practical strategies and motivational insights, Michaels has inspired countless individuals to embark on their weight loss journeys with confidence and determination.

DiNICOLANTONIO: THE OBESITY FIX

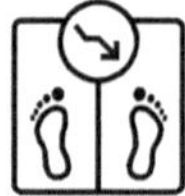

Dr. James DiNicolantonio is a well-respected cardiovascular research scientist and a Doctor of Pharmacy known for his work in nutrition and health. He has written several books, including *The Obesity Fix*. Here are the key principles Dr. DiNicolantonio emphasizes for effective and sustainable weight loss:

Understanding the Root Causes of Obesity

At the core of Dr. DiNicolantonio's approach is identifying and addressing the underlying causes of obesity. He argues that the modern diet, high in processed foods, refined carbohydrates, and added sugars, is a major driver of weight gain. Additionally, he highlights the role of hormonal imbalances, particularly insulin resistance, in promoting fat storage and making weight loss difficult.

The Importance of Insulin Regulation

Dr. DiNicolantonio places a strong emphasis on regulating insulin levels through dietary changes. He explains that high insulin levels, often caused by a diet rich in refined carbs and sugars, can lead to fat accumulation and make it challenging to lose weight. By reducing carbohydrate intake and focusing on whole, nutrient-dense foods, individuals can help lower insulin levels and optimize fat burning.

Dietary Recommendations

Dr. DiNicolantonio advocates for a diet that is low in refined carbohydrates and high in healthy fats, lean proteins, and fiber-rich vegetables. He encourages the consumption of:

- Leafy greens and non-starchy vegetables

- Lean proteins like chicken, turkey, and fish

- Healthy fats from sources such as avocados, nuts, and olive oil

- Whole, unprocessed carbohydrates like quinoa, brown rice, and berries

He discourages the intake of processed foods, added sugars, and refined carbohydrates, as they can contribute to insulin resistance and weight gain.

Mindset and Behavioral Changes

Dr. DiNicolantonio emphasizes the importance of developing a positive mindset and making sustainable behavioral changes for successful weight loss. He encourages individuals to focus on overall health rather than just aesthetics and to view weight loss as a journey rather than a quick fix. By fostering a healthy relationship with food and developing mindful eating habits, individuals can achieve lasting results.

Importance of Exercise

While diet is the primary focus, Dr. DiNicolantonio also stresses the benefits of regular physical activity for weight loss and overall health. He recommends incorporating a combination of aerobic exercise and strength training into one's routine. Exercise not only helps burn calories but also improves insulin sensitivity and supports muscle maintenance.

Addressing Emotional Eating

Recognizing the emotional aspects of eating, Dr. DiNicolantonio encourages individuals to identify their triggers for emotional eating and develop healthier coping mechanisms. This may involve seeking support from friends or professionals, practicing stress-reduction techniques, or engaging in hobbies that provide a healthy outlet for emotions.

Individualization and Sustainability

Dr. DiNicolantonio acknowledges that there is no one-size-fits-all approach to weight loss. He encourages individuals to experiment with different dietary approaches and exercise routines to find what works best for their unique needs and preferences. By focusing on long-term sustainability and making gradual changes, individuals are more likely to maintain their weight loss and enjoy the benefits of improved health.

Supplements and Micronutrients

While emphasizing the importance of obtaining nutrients from whole foods, Dr. DiNicolantonio recognizes the potential role of certain supplements in supporting weight loss and overall health.

He highlights the importance of micronutrients like magnesium, omega-3 fatty acids, and vitamin D in regulating metabolism and reducing inflammation. However, he advises consulting with a healthcare professional before starting any supplement regimen.

Foster a Positive Connection with Food

Dr. James DiNicolantonio emphasizes the importance of developing a healthier relationship with food as a cornerstone of his weight loss philosophy in *The Obesity Fix*. He believes that understanding and improving this relationship is crucial for sustainable weight loss and overall well-being. Here's a deeper exploration of his strategies to foster a positive connection with food:

1. Mindful Eating

One of the key strategies Dr. DiNicolantonio advocates is mindful eating. This involves being fully present during meals, paying attention to the flavors, textures, and aromas of food, and recognizing hunger and satiety cues. By practicing mindfulness, individuals can:

- **Slow Down:** Taking the time to savor each bite allows the body to register fullness, reducing the likelihood of overeating. Dr. DiNicolantonio suggests putting down utensils between bites and minimizing distractions, such as television or smartphones, during meals.

- **Tune into Hunger Signals:** Mindful eating encourages individuals to listen to their bodies rather than eat out of habit or emotional triggers. This self-awareness helps distinguish between true hunger and emotional or situational eating.

2. Reframing Food Choices

Dr. DiNicolantonio encourages readers to shift their mindset from viewing food as a source of guilt or restriction to seeing it as a means of nourishment and enjoyment. This involves:

- **Focusing on Nutritional Value:** Instead of counting calories or obsessing over food restrictions, individuals should prioritize foods that provide essential nutrients. This means choosing whole, unprocessed foods rich in vitamins, minerals, and fiber, which promote overall health.

- **Embracing Variety**: A diverse diet can make meals more enjoyable and satisfying. By incorporating a wide range of foods, individuals can discover new flavors and textures while ensuring they receive a broad spectrum of nutrients.

3. Understanding Emotional Eating

Recognizing the emotional aspects of eating is crucial for developing a healthier relationship with food. Dr. DiNicolantonio emphasizes the need to:

- **Identify Triggers**: Individuals should take time to reflect on their eating habits and identify situations or emotions that lead to unhealthy eating. Keeping a food diary can help track these patterns and increase self-awareness.

- **Develop Healthy Coping Mechanisms**: Instead of turning to food for comfort, Dr. DiNicolantonio encourages finding alternative ways to cope with stress or emotions. This might include engaging in physical activity, practicing relaxation techniques (like relaxation exercise or meditation), or pursuing hobbies that bring joy.

4. Eliminating Food Guilt

Dr. DiNicolantonio believes that guilt surrounding food choices can lead to unhealthy eating patterns and a negative relationship with food. He suggests:

- **Practicing Self-Compassion**: It's important to treat oneself with kindness and understanding, especially when indulging in less healthy foods. Instead of labeling foods as "good" or "bad," individuals should adopt a more balanced perspective, recognizing that occasional treats can be part of a healthy lifestyle.

- **Making Peace with Food**: By eliminating the stigma attached to certain foods, individuals can enjoy them without guilt. This mindset shift can help prevent binge eating and promote a more balanced approach to nutrition.

5. Educating Yourself About Nutrition

Dr. DiNicolantonio encourages readers to take an active role in understanding nutrition and how different foods affect their bodies. This involves:

- **Researching Nutritional Information**: Learning about the benefits of various foods and how they contribute to health can empower individuals to make informed choices. This knowledge can help them select foods that align with their health goals.

- **Consulting Professionals**: Seeking guidance from registered dietitians or nutritionists can provide personalized advice and support in developing a healthy eating plan that fits individual needs and preferences.

6. Setting Realistic Goals

Dr. DiNicolantonio emphasizes the importance of setting achievable, realistic goals related to food and weight loss. This includes:

- **Focusing on Progress, Not Perfection**: Individuals should celebrate small victories and recognize that weight loss is a journey with ups and downs. Embracing a flexible mindset allows for adjustments along the way without feeling discouraged.

- **Creating Sustainable Habits**: Rather than pursuing extreme diets or quick fixes, individuals should aim to establish long-lasting habits that promote health and well-being. This might include meal prepping, cooking at home, and planning balanced meals.

Emotional Triggers for Overeating

Dr. James DiNicolantonio emphasizes the importance of identifying emotional triggers for overeating as a key strategy for developing a healthier relationship with food and achieving sustainable weight loss. Here's a more in-depth look at this aspect of his approach:

Understanding Emotional Eating

Emotional eating refers to the tendency to turn to food, particularly unhealthy foods, as a way to cope with negative emotions or stress. Dr. DiNicolantonio recognizes that emotional eating is a common barrier to weight loss and maintaining a healthy weight. He explains that while food may provide temporary comfort or distraction, it ultimately fails to address the underlying emotional issues and can lead to feelings of guilt, shame, and further emotional distress.

Identifying Emotional Triggers

The first step in overcoming emotional eating, according to Dr. DiNicolantonio, is to identify the specific emotions and situations that trigger the urge to overeat. He encourages readers to keep a food diary or journal to track their eating habits and the emotions they experience before, during, and after eating. This self-awareness can help individuals recognize patterns and pinpoint the triggers that lead to emotional eating episodes.Common emotional triggers for overeating may include:

- Stress, anxiety, or worry

- Boredom or loneliness

- Depression or sadness

- Anger or frustration

- Feelings of low self-worth or body dissatisfaction

By becoming aware of these triggers, individuals can start to develop strategies to address the underlying emotions in healthier ways.

Developing Coping Mechanisms

Once emotional triggers have been identified, Dr. DiNicolantonio encourages readers to find alternative ways to cope with difficult emotions that do not involve food. He suggests a variety of strategies, such as:

- Practicing stress-reduction techniques like deep breathing, meditation, or relaxation exercise

- Engaging in physical activity or exercise to release tension and boost mood

- Reaching out to supportive friends or family members for emotional support

- Pursuing hobbies or activities that bring joy and a sense of accomplishment

- Seeking professional help from a therapist or counselor if needed

By developing a toolbox of healthy coping mechanisms, individuals can learn to manage their emotions without turning to food as a way to numb or escape them.

Mindful Eating

In addition to finding alternative coping strategies, Dr. DiNicolantonio emphasizes the importance of practicing mindful eating. This involves being fully present during meals, paying attention to hunger and fullness cues, and savoring the flavors and textures of food. By slowing down and being mindful, individuals can become more aware of their emotional state and make more conscious choices about what and how much they eat.

Self-Compassion and Persistence

Overcoming emotional eating is a process that requires patience, self-compassion, and persistence. Dr. DiNicolantonio encourages readers to be kind to themselves throughout the journey and to view setbacks as opportunities for learning and growth. He emphasizes that change takes time and that it's important to keep trying even when faced with challenges or slip-ups.

Motivation and Accountability

Dr. James DiNicolantonio emphasizes also the importance of maintaining motivation and accountability as crucial components of successful weight loss in his book *The Obesity Fix*. He provides several strategies to help individuals stay committed to their weight loss goals and make lasting changes. Here's a detailed look at these strategies:

1. Setting Realistic Goals

Dr. DiNicolantonio advocates for setting achievable and realistic goals rather than aiming for drastic changes. This involves:

- **Specificity**: Goals should be clear and specific. Instead of saying, "I want to lose weight," a more specific goal would be, "I want to lose 10 pounds in the next three months."

- **Measurable Outcomes**: Establishing measurable outcomes helps track progress. This could include tracking weight, body measurements, or fitness levels.

- **Time-Bound**: Setting a timeline for goals creates a sense of urgency and helps individuals stay focused.

By breaking down larger goals into smaller, manageable milestones, individuals can celebrate their achievements along the way, which boosts motivation.

2. Creating a Support System

Dr. DiNicolantonio emphasizes the importance of having a strong support system to maintain motivation. This can include:

- **Family and Friends**: Sharing weight loss goals with family and friends can create a network of support. Encouragement from loved ones can help individuals stay accountable and motivated.

- **Support Groups**: Joining a weight loss group or community, whether in-person or online, can provide additional support and motivation. Sharing experiences, challenges, and successes with others can foster a sense of camaraderie.

- **Professional Guidance**: Consulting with a registered dietitian, nutritionist, or personal trainer can provide personalized advice and accountability. Professionals can help tailor a plan that aligns with individual goals and preferences.

3. Tracking Progress

Dr. DiNicolantonio encourages individuals to actively track their progress to maintain motivation. This can involve:

- **Food Journals**: Keeping a food diary helps individuals become more aware of their eating habits and identify patterns. Writing down meals, snacks, and emotions associated with eating can provide valuable insights.

- **Regular Weigh-Ins**: While the scale is not the only indicator of progress, regular weigh-ins can help individuals stay accountable. Dr. DiNicolantonio suggests weighing in at the same time each week to monitor trends.

- **Fitness Tracking**: Using fitness apps or wearable devices to track physical activity can help individuals stay motivated to meet their exercise goals.

4. Emphasizing Non-Scale Victories

Dr. DiNicolantonio highlights the importance of recognizing non-scale victories, which can be just as motivating as weight loss. These victories might include:

- **Increased Energy Levels**: Noticing improved energy and vitality can be a significant motivator.

- **Improved Mood and Mental Clarity**: Many individuals experience enhanced mood and cognitive function as they adopt healthier habits.

- **Clothing Fit**: Feeling more comfortable in clothes or noticing changes in body shape can be encouraging.

By focusing on these non-scale victories, individuals can maintain motivation even when the scale does not reflect their efforts.

5. Building a Routine

Establishing a consistent routine can help individuals stay on track with their weight loss goals. Dr. DiNicolantonio suggests:

- **Meal Planning**: Preparing meals in advance can help individuals make healthier choices and avoid impulsive eating.

- **Scheduled Workouts**: Treating exercise like an appointment by scheduling workouts can help ensure consistency. Finding a time that works best for individual schedules can make it easier to stick to a routine.

- **Healthy Habits**: Incorporating healthy habits into daily routines, such as drinking water before meals or taking the stairs instead of the elevator, can contribute to overall progress.

6. Practicing Self-Compassion

Dr. DiNicolantonio stresses the importance of self-compassion in the weight loss journey. This involves:

- **Forgiving Setbacks**: Recognizing that setbacks are a natural part of the process can help individuals maintain motivation. Instead of being overly critical, individuals should focus on learning from their experiences.

- **Positive Self-Talk**: Encouraging positive self-talk can help combat negative thoughts that may arise during challenging times. Dr. DiNicolantonio advocates for replacing self-criticism with affirmations and supportive language.

7. Staying Educated

Finally, Dr. DiNicolantonio encourages individuals to stay informed about nutrition and health. This can involve:

- **Reading and Research**: Engaging with reputable sources of information about nutrition, exercise, and health can empower individuals to make informed choices.

- **Continuous Learning**: Attending workshops, seminars, or webinars on nutrition and wellness can provide new insights and strategies for maintaining motivation.

Changes that Help Regulate Insulin Levels

Dr. James DiNicolantonio emphasizes the importance of dietary changes that help regulate insulin levels as a crucial strategy for effective weight loss and overall health. His approach focuses on reducing carbohydrate intake and prioritizing whole foods, which can lead to improved insulin sensitivity and better metabolic health. Here's a detailed look at this strategy:

Understanding Insulin and Its Role in Weight Management

Insulin is a hormone produced by the pancreas that plays a vital role in regulating blood sugar levels.

When we consume carbohydrates, they are broken down into glucose, which enters the bloodstream. In response, the pancreas releases insulin to help cells absorb glucose for energy or store it as fat.However, when insulin levels remain chronically elevated due to a diet high in refined carbohydrates and sugars, the body can develop insulin resistance. This condition makes it more difficult for the body to use insulin effectively, leading to weight gain, increased fat storage, and a higher risk of developing type 2 diabetes and other metabolic disorders.

1. Reducing Carbohydrate Intake

Dr. DiNicolantonio advocates for reducing carbohydrate intake, particularly refined carbohydrates and sugars, as a means to lower insulin levels. Here are some key points regarding this approach:

- **Focus on Low Glycemic Index Foods**: Foods with a low glycemic index (GI) cause a slower, more gradual rise in blood sugar levels, leading to lower insulin responses. Examples include non-starchy vegetables, legumes, whole grains, and certain fruits like berries.

- **Limit Refined Carbohydrates**: Dr. DiNicolantonio advises avoiding refined carbohydrates found in white bread, pastries, sugary snacks, and soft drinks. These foods can cause rapid spikes in blood sugar and insulin levels, promoting fat storage.

- **Consider a Low-Carb Diet**: Many individuals find success with low-carb diets, which typically limit carbohydrate intake to around 20-50 grams per day. This approach encourages the body to enter a state of ketosis, where it burns fat for fuel instead of relying on carbohydrates.

2. Emphasizing Whole Foods

In addition to reducing carbohydrate intake, Dr. DiNicolantonio stresses the importance of focusing on whole, unprocessed foods. This dietary approach is beneficial for several reasons:

- **Nutrient Density**: Whole foods, such as fruits, vegetables, lean proteins, nuts, seeds, and healthy fats, are rich in essential nutrients, vitamins, and minerals. These foods provide the body with the necessary building blocks for optimal health and metabolic function.

- **Fiber-Rich Foods**: Whole foods are often high in dietary fiber, which can help regulate blood sugar levels by slowing the absorption of glucose into the bloodstream. Fiber also promotes satiety, reducing the likelihood of overeating.

- **Healthy Fats**: Incorporating healthy fats from sources like avocados, olive oil, nuts, and fatty fish can help improve insulin sensitivity. Fats can provide a feeling of fullness and satisfaction, making it easier to adhere to a lower carbohydrate diet.

3. Meal Composition and Timing

Dr. DiNicolantonio emphasizes the importance of meal composition and timing in regulating insulin levels:

- **Balanced Meals**: Each meal should include a combination of lean protein, healthy fats, and low-glycemic carbohydrates. This balance helps stabilize blood sugar levels and promotes sustained energy throughout the day.

- **Regular Meal Timing**: Eating at regular intervals can help maintain stable blood sugar levels. Dr. DiNicolantonio suggests consuming smaller, more frequent meals to prevent extreme fluctuations in insulin and blood sugar.

- **Avoiding Snacking on High-Carb Foods**: Instead of reaching for high-carb snacks, individuals should opt for nutrient-dense options that include protein and healthy fats, such as nuts, yogurt, or vegetables with hummus.

4. Hydration and Insulin Sensitivity

Dr. DiNicolantonio also highlights the role of hydration in maintaining insulin sensitivity:

- **Drink Water**: Staying well-hydrated is essential for overall health and metabolic function. Drinking water can help regulate appetite and prevent confusion between thirst and hunger.

- **Limit Sugary Beverages**: Sugary drinks can lead to rapid spikes in blood sugar and insulin levels. Dr. DiNicolantonio recommends avoiding sodas, fruit juices, and other sweetened beverages in favor of water, herbal teas, or black coffee.

5. Monitoring Progress and Adjusting Diet

Finally, Dr. DiNicolantonio encourages individuals to monitor their progress and make adjustments to their diets as needed:

- **Track Food Intake**: Keeping a food diary can help individuals become more aware of their carbohydrate intake and overall eating patterns. This awareness can lead to more informed choices.

- **Listen to Your Body**: Paying attention to how different foods affect energy levels, mood, and hunger can provide valuable insights into what works best for each individual.

- **Consult with Professionals**: Working with a registered dietitian or nutritionist can provide personalized guidance and support in developing a low-carb, whole-foods-based diet that meets individual health goals.

Conclusion

Dr. James DiNicolantonio's approach to weight loss, as outlined in "The Obesity Fix", is grounded in scientific evidence and emphasizes the importance of addressing the root causes of obesity. By focusing on insulin regulation, healthy dietary choices, regular exercise, and sustainable behavioral changes, individuals can achieve lasting weight loss and improve their overall health. Dr. DiNicolantonio's expertise in cardiovascular research and his commitment to evidence-based solutions make his strategies a valuable resource for anyone seeking to lose weight and maintain a healthy lifestyle.

Identifying and addressing emotional triggers for overeating is a crucial aspect of Dr. James DiNicolantonio's approach to weight loss and overall health. By developing self-awareness, finding alternative coping mechanisms, practicing mindful eating, and cultivating self-compassion, individuals can break free from the cycle of emotional eating and develop a healthier, more sustainable relationship with food. This holistic approach empowers readers to take control of their health and well-being while enjoying the foods they love in moderation.

DiNicolantonio's strategies for maintaining motivation and accountability in weight loss are grounded in practical, evidence-based approaches. By setting realistic goals, creating a support system, tracking progress, emphasizing non-scale victories, building routines, practicing self-compassion, and staying educated, individuals can foster a sustainable and motivating environment for their weight loss journey. These strategies not only help individuals achieve their weight loss goals but also promote a healthier, more balanced lifestyle overall.

Dr. James DiNicolantonio's approach to weight loss emphasizes the importance of dietary changes that regulate insulin levels through reducing carbohydrate intake and focusing on whole foods. By adopting these strategies, individuals can improve their metabolic health, promote fat loss, and develop a healthier relationship with food. This holistic approach not only supports weight loss but also fosters long-term health and well-being.

HORTON: P90X WORKOUT PROGRAM

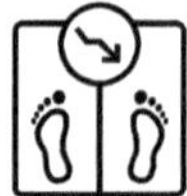

Tony Horton, the creator of the popular P90X workout program, has developed a holistic approach to weight loss that emphasizes consistent exercise, balanced nutrition, and a positive mindset. His philosophy is rooted in the belief that fitness should be a sustainable lifestyle rather than a temporary fix. Here's an in-depth look at Horton's strategies for losing weight effectively.

1. Consistency is Key

Horton stresses that consistency is one of the most critical factors in achieving and maintaining weight loss. He believes that individuals should commit to a regular workout routine, aiming for a mix of strength training, cardio, and flexibility exercises. Horton often says, "Be the tortoise, not the hare," emphasizing that slow and steady progress is more sustainable than quick, drastic changes.

- **Regular Workouts**: Horton recommends exercising at least six days a week, incorporating a variety of activities to prevent boredom and promote overall fitness. His workouts often include strength training, relaxation exercises, and high-intensity interval training (HIIT).

- **Daily Movement**: Beyond structured workouts, Horton encourages people to integrate physical activity into their daily routines. This can include walking, gardening, or playing sports, which helps maintain a higher level of activity throughout the day.

2. Balanced Nutrition

Horton emphasizes the importance of a well-rounded diet in conjunction with exercise for effective weight loss. He advocates for a balanced intake of macronutrients—proteins, carbohydrates, and fats—while focusing on whole, unprocessed foods.

- **Whole Foods**: Horton encourages consuming nutrient-dense foods, such as fruits, vegetables, whole grains, lean proteins, and healthy fats. He believes that these foods provide the necessary vitamins and minerals to support overall health and energy levels.

- **Minimize Sugar and Processed Foods**: Horton has spoken about the negative effects of sugar on the body and encourages reducing sugar intake significantly. He advocates for avoiding processed foods that are high in added sugars and unhealthy fats.

- **Hydration**: Staying hydrated is another crucial aspect of Horton's dietary recommendations. He suggests drinking plenty of water throughout the day to support metabolism and overall health.

3. Mindfulness and Mental Attitude

Horton believes that a positive mindset plays a vital role in successful weight loss. He encourages individuals to adopt a mindful approach to their fitness journey.

- **Set Realistic Goals**: Horton advises setting achievable, realistic goals rather than aiming for drastic changes. This helps maintain motivation and reduces the likelihood of disappointment.

- **Focus on the Process**: Instead of fixating on the end result, Horton emphasizes the importance of enjoying the journey. He encourages individuals to appreciate the small victories and improvements in strength, endurance, and overall well-being.

- **Self-Compassion**: Recognizing that setbacks are a natural part of the process is essential. Horton promotes self-compassion and encourages individuals to be kind to themselves, especially during challenging times.

4. Creating a Structured Plan

Horton stresses the importance of having a structured plan for workouts and meals. This helps individuals stay accountable and organized in their weight loss efforts.

- **Workout Schedule**: Horton recommends creating a weekly workout schedule that outlines specific exercises and activities. This helps individuals commit to their fitness routine and ensures they are incorporating a variety of workouts.

- **Meal Planning**: Planning meals in advance can help individuals make healthier choices and avoid impulsive eating. Horton suggests preparing meals that include a balance of macronutrients to support energy levels and recovery.

5. Accountability and Support

Having a support system can significantly enhance motivation and adherence to a weight loss plan. Horton encourages individuals to seek accountability through various means.

- **Workout Buddies**: Exercising with friends or family members can make workouts more enjoyable and provide mutual support. Horton believes that sharing fitness goals with others can help maintain motivation.

- **Online Communities**: Joining online fitness communities or social media groups can provide additional encouragement and accountability. Engaging with others who share similar goals can foster a sense of camaraderie.

6. Incorporating Recovery

Horton emphasizes that recovery is just as important as the workout itself. Proper recovery allows the body to heal and rebuild, which is essential for long-term success.

- **Rest Days**: Incorporating rest days into the workout schedule is crucial for preventing burnout and injury. Horton recommends listening to the body and allowing time for recovery.

- **Mindfulness Practices**: Horton has integrated mindfulness practices, such as meditation and relaxation exercises, into his routine. These practices can help reduce stress and promote mental clarity, which are beneficial for overall health.

7. Embracing Variety

To prevent plateaus and maintain interest in workouts, Horton advocates for incorporating variety into exercise routines.

- **Different Workouts**: Horton encourages trying different types of workouts, such as HIIT, strength training, relaxation exercises and outdoor activities. This not only keeps workouts exciting but also challenges the body in new ways.

- **Adjusting Intensity**: Horton emphasizes that intensity can vary from day to day. It's essential to listen to the body and adjust the intensity of workouts based on energy levels and overall well-being.

Training philosophy

According to Tony Horton's training philosophy, he recommends exercising at least six days a week, incorporating a variety of activities to challenge the body and prevent plateaus. Here are some examples of exercises and workouts that Horton often includes in his programs:

Strength Training

Horton emphasizes the importance of strength training, typically dedicating three days a week to lifting weights. His strength training workouts often include:

- Compound exercises like squats, deadlifts, and bench presses to work multiple muscle groups simultaneously

- Isolation exercises to target specific muscle groups like biceps, triceps, and shoulders

- Use of resistance bands and Tonal's dynamic weight modes to add variety and challenge the muscles in new ways

Relaxing exercises

Horton dedicates one day a week to relaxing exercises, focusing on flexibility, mobility, and balance.

- Sun exercises to warm up the body

- Standing poses to build strength and stability

- Backbends and forward folds to stretch the spine

- Balancing poses to challenge proprioception

- Restorative poses for recovery

Outdoor Activities

The remaining two days of the week are spent engaging in various outdoor exercises and activities, such as:

- Climbing ropes and parallel bars for an added challenge

- Sprinting and interval training to improve cardiovascular fitness

- Bodyweight exercises like push-ups, pull-ups, and burpees

- Agility drills using cones or other equipment

Full-Body Workouts

In addition to targeted strength training and relaxation exercise, Horton incorporates full-body workouts that challenge multiple muscle groups simultaneously. These workouts often include:

- Compound exercises like squat-to-overhead presses

- Plyometric exercises like jumping lunges and box jumps

- Metabolic conditioning circuits to keep the heart rate elevated

- Bodyweight exercises that can be done anywhere

Recovery and Mobility

While Horton emphasizes the importance of consistent exercise, he also stresses the need for adequate recovery and mobility work. Some examples of recovery and mobility exercises he incorporates include:

- Foam rolling and self-myofascial release techniques

- Stretching and mobility drills to improve range of motion

- Epsom salt baths to reduce muscle soreness and inflammation

- Meditation and breathwork to manage stress and promote relaxation

By incorporating a variety of exercises and activities into his training plans, Horton aims to keep workouts engaging, challenging, and effective for overall fitness and weight loss. The key is finding a balance between pushing hard and allowing the body to recover, ultimately creating a sustainable fitness routine that can be maintained for the long term.

Conclusion

Tony Horton's approach to weight loss is comprehensive and emphasizes the importance of consistency, balanced nutrition, mindfulness, and support. By focusing on sustainable lifestyle changes rather than quick fixes, individuals can achieve lasting results. Horton's philosophy encourages a positive mindset, structured planning, and the incorporation of variety into workouts, making fitness an enjoyable and integral part of life. Through his guidance, many have found success in their weight loss journeys, proving that with dedication and the right strategies, achieving fitness goals is possible for everyone.

RELAXATION EXERCISES

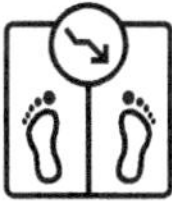

Relaxation exercises are an effective way to reduce stress, improve overall well-being, and promote better sleep. While yoga is a popular form of relaxation, there are several other techniques that can be practiced without the need for yoga. In this text, we will explore various relaxation exercises that can be done easily and conveniently, regardless of your fitness level or experience.

It is better to find alternatives to yoga, because yoga is often used to cover over deeper mental and spiritual problems. Yoga hide them, but not solve them.

It should not be forgotten that yoga originated in Hinduism, which is characterised by various practices that are also directed against some groups of people. This spiritual system includes issues like contempt for people of lower castes.

Deep Breathing Exercises

Deep breathing is one of the simplest and most effective relaxation techniques. It helps activate the parasympathetic nervous system, which is responsible for the body's rest and digest response. Here are a few deep breathing exercises to try:

1. **Diaphragmatic breathing**: Lie down or sit comfortably, placing one hand on your belly and the other on your chest. Inhale slowly through your nose, feeling your belly rise. Exhale slowly through your mouth, feeling your belly fall. Repeat for several minutes.

2. **4-7-8 breathing**: Inhale for 4 seconds, hold your breath for 7 seconds, and exhale for 8 seconds. Repeat this cycle several times.

3. **Alternate nostril breathing**: Close your right nostril with your thumb and inhale through your left nostril. Close your left nostril with your index finger and exhale through your right nostril. Repeat, alternating nostrils.

Progressive Muscle Relaxation

Progressive muscle relaxation (PMR) involves systematically tensing and releasing different muscle groups throughout the body. This technique helps you become more aware of physical tension and how to release it. Here's how to practice PMR:

1. Sit or lie down in a comfortable position.

2. Focus on one muscle group at a time, such as your feet or hands.

3. Inhale and tense the muscles in that group for 5-10 seconds.

4. Exhale and quickly release the tension, letting the muscles relax.

5. Repeat with each muscle group, working your way up or down your body.

Visualization and Guided Imagery

Visualization and guided imagery involve creating mental images of peaceful, calming scenes or experiences. This technique can help shift your focus away from stressful thoughts and promote a sense of relaxation. Here's how to practice visualization:

1. Find a quiet, comfortable place to sit or lie down.

2. Close your eyes and take a few deep breaths.

3. Imagine a peaceful, calming scene, such as a beach, forest, or mountain. Use all your senses to make the image as vivid as possible.

4. Focus on the details of your chosen scene, such as the colors, sounds, and smells.

5. If your mind wanders, gently bring your attention back to the visualization.

Mindfulness Meditation

Mindfulness meditation involves focusing your attention on the present moment, without judgment or criticism. This technique can help reduce stress, improve focus, and promote a sense of calm. Here's how to practice mindfulness meditation:

1. Find a quiet, comfortable place to sit.

2. Close your eyes and focus on your breathing, noticing the sensation of air moving in and out of your body.

3. When your mind wanders, gently bring your attention back to your breath.

4. If you notice any thoughts or feelings, acknowledge them without judgment and return your focus to your breath.

5. Start with just a few minutes per day and gradually increase the duration as you become more comfortable with the practice.

Conclusion

Relaxation exercises are a powerful tool for reducing stress, improving sleep, and promoting overall well-being. By incorporating deep breathing, progressive muscle relaxation, visualization, and mindfulness meditation into your daily routine, you can cultivate a greater sense of calm and resilience in the face of life's challenges. Remember, finding the right relaxation technique for you may take some experimentation, but the benefits are well worth the effort.

BREAKFAST RECIPES

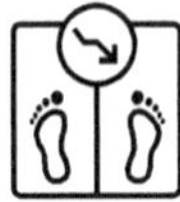

Here are 15 healthy breakfast recipes that support weight loss, emphasizing high protein, fiber, and healthy fats. These options are designed to keep you full and energized throughout the morning while helping you achieve your weight loss goals.

1. Egg Muffins

Ingredients:

- 6 large eggs

- 1 cup chopped vegetables (spinach, bell peppers, onions)

- 1/2 cup shredded cheese (optional)

- Salt and pepper to taste

Instructions:

1. Preheat the oven to 350°F (175°C).

2. Whisk the eggs in a bowl and season with salt and pepper.

3. Stir in the chopped vegetables and cheese.

4. Pour the mixture into a greased muffin tin.

5. Bake for 20-25 minutes or until set. Let cool and store in the fridge for a quick breakfast.

2. Greek Yogurt with Berries and Chia Seeds

Ingredients:

- 1 cup Greek yogurt

- 1/2 cup mixed berries (blueberries, strawberries)

- 1 tablespoon chia seeds

- Honey or maple syrup (optional)

Instructions:

1. In a bowl, combine Greek yogurt, berries, and chia seeds.

2. Drizzle with honey or maple syrup if desired. Enjoy immediately.

3. Peanut Butter Oats

Ingredients:

- 1/2 cup rolled oats

- 1 cup almond milk (or any milk of choice)

- 2 tablespoons peanut butter

- 1 banana, sliced

- Cinnamon to taste

Instructions:

1. In a saucepan, combine oats and almond milk. Cook over medium heat until thickened.

2. Stir in peanut butter and cinnamon.

3. Top with banana slices before serving.

4. Breakfast Burrito

Ingredients:

- 1 whole grain tortilla

- 2 scrambled eggs

- 1/4 avocado, sliced

- 1/4 cup black beans

- Salsa to taste

Instructions:

1. Scramble the eggs in a pan.

2. Place the scrambled eggs, avocado, black beans, and salsa on the tortilla.

3. Roll up the tortilla and enjoy.

5. Chia Seed Pudding

Ingredients:

- 1/4 cup chia seeds

- 1 cup almond milk (or any milk of choice)

- 1 tablespoon maple syrup or honey

- Fresh fruit for topping

Instructions:

1. In a bowl, mix chia seeds, almond milk, and sweetener.

2. Stir well and refrigerate overnight.

3. In the morning, top with fresh fruit before serving.

6. Avocado Toast with Poached Eggs

Ingredients:

- 1 slice whole grain bread

- 1/2 avocado

- 2 poached eggs

- Salt, pepper, and red pepper flakes to taste

Instructions:

1. Toast the bread and mash the avocado on top.

2. Poach the eggs and place them on the avocado toast.

3. Season with salt, pepper, and red pepper flakes.

7. Smoothie Bowl

Ingredients:

- 1 banana

- 1/2 cup spinach

- 1/2 cup almond milk

- 1 tablespoon almond butter

- Toppings: granola, sliced fruit, nuts

Instructions:

1. Blend the banana, spinach, almond milk, and almond butter until smooth.

2. Pour into a bowl and top with granola and sliced fruit.

8. Quinoa Breakfast Bowl

Ingredients:

- 1/2 cup cooked quinoa

- 1/2 cup almond milk

- 1 tablespoon maple syrup

- 1/4 cup mixed berries

- 1 tablespoon nuts or seeds

Instructions:

1. In a bowl, combine cooked quinoa, almond milk, and maple syrup.

2. Top with berries and nuts before serving.

9. Overnight Oats

Ingredients:

- 1/2 cup rolled oats

- 1/2 cup almond milk

- 1 tablespoon chia seeds

- 1/2 banana, sliced

- Cinnamon to taste

Instructions:

1. In a jar, combine oats, almond milk, chia seeds, and cinnamon.

2. Stir well and refrigerate overnight.

3. Top with banana slices before eating.

10. Tofu Scramble

Ingredients:

- 1 block firm tofu, crumbled

- 1 cup spinach

- 1/2 bell pepper, diced

- 1 tablespoon nutritional yeast

- Salt and pepper to taste

Instructions:

1. In a pan, sauté bell pepper until soft.

2. Add crumbled tofu and spinach, cooking until heated through.

3. Stir in nutritional yeast and season with salt and pepper.

11. Healthy Breakfast Casserole

Ingredients:

- 6 large eggs

- 1 cup chopped vegetables (zucchini, bell peppers, onions)

- 1/2 cup low-fat cheese

- Salt and pepper to taste

Instructions:

1. Preheat the oven to 350°F (175°C).

2. Whisk eggs in a bowl and add vegetables and cheese.

3. Pour into a greased baking dish and bake for 25-30 minutes until set.

12. Berry Protein Smoothie

Ingredients:

- 1 cup mixed berries (fresh or frozen)

- 1 scoop protein powder

- 1 cup spinach

- 1 cup almond milk

Instructions:

1. Blend all ingredients until smooth.

2. Pour into a glass and enjoy as a quick breakfast.

13. Egg and Vegetable Frittata

Ingredients:

- 6 large eggs

- 1 cup mixed vegetables (spinach, tomatoes, mushrooms)

- 1/2 cup feta cheese

- Salt and pepper to taste

Instructions:

1. Preheat the oven to 375°F (190°C).

2. Whisk eggs and season with salt and pepper.

3. Mix in vegetables and feta cheese, pour into a greased baking dish.

4. Bake for 25-30 minutes until set.

14. Cottage Cheese with Fruit and Nuts

Ingredients:

- 1 cup cottage cheese

- 1/2 cup pineapple or berries

- 1 tablespoon chopped nuts (almonds or walnuts)

Instructions:

1. In a bowl, combine cottage cheese with fruit and top with nuts.

2. Enjoy as a quick and nutritious breakfast.

15. Oatmeal with Almond Butter and Banana

Ingredients:

- 1/2 cup rolled oats

- 1 cup water or almond milk

- 1 tablespoon almond butter

- 1 banana, sliced

- Cinnamon to taste

Instructions:

1. Cook oats in water or almond milk according to package instructions.

2. Stir in almond butter and top with banana slices and cinnamon.

These recipes are designed to provide a nutritious start to your day, helping you feel full and satisfied while supporting your weight loss journey. Enjoy experimenting with these options to find your favorites!

LUNCH RECIPES

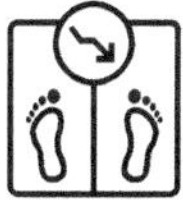

Here are 15 healthy lunch recipes designed to support weight loss. These meals are balanced, nutritious, and packed with flavor, helping you stay satisfied and energized throughout the day.

1. Grilled Chicken Salad

Ingredients:

- 4 oz grilled chicken breast, sliced

- 2 cups mixed greens (spinach, arugula, romaine)

- 1/2 cup cherry tomatoes, halved

- 1/4 cucumber, sliced

- 2 tablespoons vinaigrette dressing

Instructions:

1. In a large bowl, combine mixed greens, cherry tomatoes, and cucumber.

2. Top with grilled chicken and drizzle with vinaigrette. Toss gently and serve.

2. Quinoa and Black Bean Bowl

Ingredients:

- 1 cup cooked quinoa

- 1/2 cup canned black beans, rinsed and drained

- 1/2 avocado, diced

- 1/2 cup corn (fresh or frozen)

- Salsa to taste

Instructions:

1. In a bowl, combine quinoa, black beans, avocado, and corn.

2. Top with salsa and mix well before serving.

3. Turkey and Spinach Wrap

Ingredients:

- 1 whole grain tortilla

- 4 oz sliced turkey breast

- 1 cup fresh spinach

- 1/4 avocado, sliced

- Mustard or hummus for spreading

Instructions:

1. Spread mustard or hummus on the tortilla.

2. Layer turkey, spinach, and avocado on top.

3. Roll up tightly and slice in half.

4. Lentil Soup

Ingredients:

- 1 cup cooked lentils

- 1 cup vegetable broth

- 1/2 cup diced carrots

- 1/2 cup diced celery

- 1/2 onion, chopped

- Salt and pepper to taste

Instructions:

1. In a pot, sauté onion, carrots, and celery until softened.

2. Add cooked lentils and vegetable broth. Simmer for 15 minutes.

3. Season with salt and pepper before serving.

5. Mediterranean Chickpea Salad

Ingredients:

- 1 can chickpeas, rinsed and drained

- 1/2 cup diced cucumber

- 1/2 cup cherry tomatoes, halved

- 1/4 red onion, diced

- 2 tablespoons olive oil

- 1 tablespoon lemon juice

- Salt and pepper to taste

Instructions:

1. In a bowl, combine chickpeas, cucumber, tomatoes, and red onion.

2. Drizzle with olive oil and lemon juice. Season with salt and pepper, then toss to combine.

6. Zucchini Noodles with Pesto

Ingredients:

- 2 medium zucchinis, spiralized

- 1/4 cup pesto

- 1/2 cup cherry tomatoes, halved

- 2 tablespoons grated Parmesan cheese (optional)

Instructions:

1. In a skillet, lightly sauté zucchini noodles for 2-3 minutes.

2. Remove from heat and toss with pesto and cherry tomatoes.

3. Top with Parmesan cheese if desired.

7. Spicy Tuna Salad

Ingredients:

- 1 can tuna, drained

- 2 tablespoons Greek yogurt

- 1 tablespoon sriracha (or to taste)

- 1/4 cup diced celery

- Salt and pepper to taste

Instructions:

1. In a bowl, combine tuna, Greek yogurt, sriracha, and celery.

2. Season with salt and pepper. Serve on whole grain bread or lettuce wraps.

8. Egg and Avocado Toast

Ingredients:

- 1 slice whole grain bread, toasted

- 1/2 avocado, mashed

- 1 hard-boiled egg, sliced

- Salt, pepper, and red pepper flakes to taste

Instructions:

1. Spread mashed avocado on the toasted bread.

2. Top with sliced hard-boiled egg and season with salt, pepper, and red pepper flakes.

9. Cauliflower Fried Rice

Ingredients:

- 2 cups cauliflower rice

- 1/2 cup mixed vegetables (peas, carrots, corn)

- 1 egg, beaten

- 2 tablespoons soy sauce

- Green onions for garnish

Instructions:

1. In a skillet, sauté cauliflower rice and mixed vegetables until tender.

2. Push to the side and scramble the egg in the pan. Mix everything together.

3. Add soy sauce and garnish with green onions before serving.

10. Shrimp and Avocado Salad

Ingredients:

- 4 oz cooked shrimp

- 1/2 avocado, diced

- 2 cups mixed greens

- 1/4 cup diced red onion

- 2 tablespoons lime juice

Instructions:

1. In a bowl, combine shrimp, avocado, mixed greens, and red onion.

2. Drizzle with lime juice and toss gently before serving.

11. Sweet Potato and Black Bean Tacos

Ingredients:

- 1 medium sweet potato, diced and roasted

- 1/2 cup canned black beans, rinsed and drained

- Corn tortillas

- Avocado and salsa for topping

Instructions:

1. Roast sweet potato in the oven at 400°F (200°C) for 25 minutes.

2. Warm corn tortillas and fill with roasted sweet potato and black beans.

3. Top with avocado and salsa.

12. Grilled Vegetable Quinoa Salad

Ingredients:

- 1 cup cooked quinoa

- 1 cup grilled vegetables (zucchini, bell peppers, eggplant)

- 2 tablespoons balsamic vinaigrette

- Fresh basil for garnish

Instructions:

1. In a bowl, combine quinoa and grilled vegetables.

2. Drizzle with balsamic vinaigrette and toss to combine. Garnish with fresh basil.

13. Caprese Salad with Chicken

Ingredients:

- 4 oz grilled chicken breast, sliced

- 1 cup cherry tomatoes, halved

- 1/2 cup fresh mozzarella balls

- Fresh basil leaves

- Balsamic glaze for drizzling

Instructions:

1. In a bowl, layer chicken, cherry tomatoes, mozzarella, and basil.

2. Drizzle with balsamic glaze before serving.

14. Veggie-Packed Hummus Wrap

Ingredients:

- 1 whole grain tortilla

- 1/4 cup hummus

- 1/2 cup mixed vegetables (carrots, cucumbers, bell peppers)

- Spinach leaves

Instructions:

1. Spread hummus on the tortilla.

2. Layer mixed vegetables and spinach on top.

3. Roll up tightly and slice in half.

15. Baked Falafel with Tzatziki

Ingredients:

- 1 can chickpeas, rinsed and drained

- 1/4 cup chopped parsley

- 2 tablespoons flour

- 1 teaspoon cumin

- Salt and pepper to taste

- Tzatziki sauce for serving

Instructions:

1. Preheat the oven to 375°F (190°C).

2. In a food processor, combine chickpeas, parsley, flour, cumin, salt, and pepper. Blend until smooth.

3. Form into small patties and place on a baking sheet. Bake for 20-25 minutes until golden.

4. Serve with tzatziki sauce.

These lunch recipes are designed to be nutritious, satisfying, and supportive of your weight loss goals. Enjoy experimenting with these options to keep your meals exciting and healthy!

DINNER RECIPES

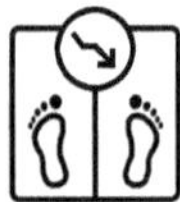

Here are 15 healthy dinner recipes that can support weight loss:

1. Baked Salmon with Roasted Vegetables

Ingredients:

- 4 oz salmon fillet

- 1 cup mixed roasted vegetables (broccoli, bell peppers, zucchini)

- 1 tbsp olive oil

- Salt and pepper to taste

Instructions:

1. Preheat oven to 400°F (200°C).

2. Toss the vegetables with olive oil, salt, and pepper. Roast for 20 minutes.

3. Season the salmon with salt and pepper. Bake for 15 minutes or until cooked through.

4. Serve the salmon with the roasted vegetables.

2. Zucchini Noodles with Turkey Meatballs

Ingredients:

- 2 cups spiralized zucchini noodles

- 4 turkey meatballs

- 1 cup marinara sauce

- Parmesan cheese (optional)

Instructions:

1. Sauté the zucchini noodles in a pan for 2-3 minutes until tender.

2. Add the turkey meatballs and marinara sauce. Heat through.

3. Serve the zucchini noodles and meatballs topped with Parmesan cheese.

3. Grilled Chicken and Vegetable Skewers

Ingredients:

- 4 oz grilled chicken breast, cubed

- 1 cup mixed vegetables (bell peppers, onions, mushrooms, zucchini)

- 1 tbsp olive oil

- Salt and pepper to taste

Instructions:

1. Thread the chicken and vegetables onto skewers.

2. Brush with olive oil and season with salt and pepper.

3. Grill the skewers for 10-15 minutes, turning occasionally, until the chicken is cooked through and the vegetables are tender.

4. Stuffed Bell Peppers

Ingredients:

- 2 bell peppers, halved and seeded

- 1/2 cup cooked quinoa

- 1/4 cup black beans, rinsed and drained

- 2 tbsp salsa

- 2 tbsp shredded cheese (optional)

Instructions:

1. Preheat oven to 375°F (190°C).

2. In a bowl, mix the quinoa, black beans, and salsa.

3. Stuff the bell pepper halves with the quinoa mixture.

4. Place the stuffed peppers in a baking dish and bake for 20 minutes.

5. Top with shredded cheese if desired and bake for an additional 5 minutes.

5. Lentil and Sweet Potato Curry

Ingredients:

- 1 cup cooked lentils

- 1 cup diced sweet potatoes

- 1 cup coconut milk

- 1 tbsp curry powder

- Salt and pepper to taste

Instructions:

1. In a saucepan, combine the lentils, sweet potatoes, coconut milk, and curry powder.

2. Simmer for 15-20 minutes, stirring occasionally, until the sweet potatoes are tender.

3. Season with salt and pepper to taste.

6. Shrimp Scampi with Zucchini Noodles

Ingredients:

- 4 oz shrimp, peeled and deveined

- 2 cups spiralized zucchini noodles

- 2 tbsp butter

- 2 cloves garlic, minced

- 1/4 cup white wine (optional)

- Salt and pepper to taste

Instructions:

1. In a skillet, melt the butter over medium heat. Add the garlic and sauté for 1 minute.

2. Add the shrimp and white wine (if using). Cook for 2-3 minutes until the shrimp are pink and opaque.

3. Add the zucchini noodles and toss to combine. Cook for an additional 2 minutes.

4. Season with salt and pepper to taste.

7. Baked Chicken Parmesan with Zucchini Noodles

Ingredients:

- 4 oz chicken breast, pounded thin

- 1/4 cup breadcrumbs

- 2 tbsp grated Parmesan cheese

- 1 egg, beaten

- 1 cup marinara sauce

- 2 cups spiralized zucchini noodles

Instructions:

1. Preheat oven to 400°F (200°C).

2. In a shallow dish, mix the breadcrumbs and Parmesan cheese.

3. Dip the chicken in the beaten egg, then coat with the breadcrumb mixture.

4. Place the breaded chicken on a baking sheet and bake for 20 minutes.

5. Top the chicken with marinara sauce and bake for an additional 5 minutes.

6. Serve the chicken parmesan over zucchini noodles.

8. Beef and Broccoli Stir-Fry

Ingredients:

- 4 oz lean beef, sliced

- 2 cups broccoli florets

- 1 tbsp soy sauce

- 1 tsp sesame oil

- 1 clove garlic, minced

- 1 tsp cornstarch

- Salt and pepper to taste

Instructions:

1. In a bowl, mix the soy sauce, sesame oil, garlic, and cornstarch.

2. Add the beef and toss to coat.

3. In a skillet, stir-fry the beef for 2-3 minutes until browned.

4. Add the broccoli and stir-fry for an additional 3-4 minutes until the broccoli is tender-crisp.

5. Season with salt and pepper to taste.

9. Baked Cod with Roasted Brussels Sprouts

Ingredients:

- 4 oz cod fillet

- 1 cup Brussels sprouts, halved

- 1 tbsp olive oil

- Salt and pepper to taste

Instructions:

1. Preheat oven to 400°F (200°C).

2. Toss the Brussels sprouts with olive oil, salt, and pepper. Roast for 20 minutes.

3. Season the cod with salt and pepper. Bake for 15 minutes or until cooked through.

4. Serve the baked cod with the roasted Brussels sprouts.

10. Grilled Chicken Caesar Salad

Ingredients:

- 4 oz grilled chicken breast, sliced

- 2 cups romaine lettuce, chopped

- 1/4 cup croutons

- 2 tbsp grated Parmesan cheese

- 2 tbsp Caesar dressing

Instructions:

1. In a large bowl, combine the romaine lettuce, grilled chicken, croutons, and Parmesan cheese.

2. Drizzle with Caesar dressing and toss to coat.

11. Spaghetti Squash with Turkey Meatballs

Ingredients:

- 1 cup cooked spaghetti squash

- 4 turkey meatballs

- 1/2 cup marinara sauce

- 2 tbsp grated Parmesan cheese (optional)

Instructions:

1. In a bowl, combine the cooked spaghetti squash and marinara sauce.

2. Top with turkey meatballs and Parmesan cheese (if using).

12. Chicken and Vegetable Stir-Fry

Ingredients:

- 4 oz chicken breast, sliced

- 1 cup mixed vegetables (broccoli, bell peppers, snow peas)

- 1 tbsp soy sauce

- 1 tsp sesame oil

- 1 clove garlic, minced

- 1 tsp cornstarch

- Salt and pepper to taste

Instructions:

1. In a bowl, mix the soy sauce, sesame oil, garlic, and cornstarch.

2. Add the chicken and toss to coat.

3. In a skillet, stir-fry the chicken for 2-3 minutes until browned.

4. Add the mixed vegetables and stir-fry for an additional 3-4 minutes until the vegetables are tender-crisp.

5. Season with salt and pepper to taste.

13. Baked Tilapia with Roasted Sweet Potatoes

Ingredients:

- 4 oz tilapia fillet

- 1 cup diced sweet potatoes

- 1 tbsp olive oil

- Salt and pepper to taste

Instructions:

1. Preheat oven to 400°F (200°C).

2. Toss the sweet potatoes with olive oil, salt, and pepper. Roast for 20 minutes.

3. Season the tilapia with salt and pepper. Bake for 15 minutes or until cooked through.

4. Serve the baked tilapia with the roasted sweet potatoes.

14. Grilled Shrimp and Vegetable Skewers

Ingredients:

- 4 oz shrimp, peeled and deveined

- 1 cup mixed vegetables (zucchini, bell peppers, onions)

- 1 tbsp olive oil

- Salt and pepper to taste

Instructions:

1. Thread the shrimp and vegetables onto skewers.

2. Brush with olive oil and season with salt and pepper.

3. Grill the skewers for 10-15 minutes, turning occasionally, until the shrimp are cooked through and the vegetables are tender.

15. Baked Chicken and Broccoli Alfredo

Ingredients:

- 4 oz chicken breast, cubed

- 1 cup broccoli florets

- 1/2 cup low-fat alfredo sauce

- 2 tbsp grated Parmesan cheese

Instructions:

1. Preheat oven to 400°F (200°C).

2. In a baking dish, combine the chicken, broccoli, and alfredo sauce. Mix well.

3. Sprinkle with Parmesan cheese.

4. Bake for 20-25 minutes until the chicken is cooked through and the broccoli is tender.

These dinner recipes are designed to be nutritious, satisfying, and supportive of your weight loss goals. They incorporate a balance of lean proteins, vegetables, healthy fats, and complex carbohydrates to keep you feeling full and energized. Enjoy experimenting with these options to find your new favorite healthy dinners!

ENDNOTES

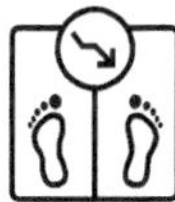

Recent advancements in obesity research highlight significant gaps between scientific findings and their application in clinical practice.

Research is exploring innovative interventions such as digital technology and telemedicine to enhance obesity treatment. Additionally, approaches like "Food Is Medicine," which includes medically tailored meals, are being investigated to prevent and treat obesity-related diseases. This highlights a shift towards integrating nutrition and health care more effectively.

There is a recognized need for more research into the cost-effectiveness of obesity prevention strategies and the long-term health outcomes of established therapies.

Collaborative efforts among researchers, healthcare providers, and policymakers are essential to bridge the gap between obesity science and practical applications in healthcare settings.

In summary, while there is a growing body of research on obesity, translating these findings into effective clinical practice remains a significant challenge. Addressing disparities, fostering innovative treatment approaches, and conducting further research are critical for advancing the field and improving outcomes for individuals affected by obesity.

REFERENCES

Ubell, Katrina. *How to Lose Weight for the Last Time: Brain-Based Solutions for Permanent Weight Loss.* New York, Grand Central Publishing, 2022.

Ubell, Katrina. *If I Am So Smart, Why Can't I Lose Weight?* [Publisher information not provided in search results], 2006.

Greger, Michael. *How Not to Die: Discover the Foods Scientifically Proven to Prevent and Reverse Disease.* New York, Flatiron Books, 2015.

Greger, Michael. *How Not to Age: The Scientific Approach to Getting Healthier as You Get Older.* New York, Flatiron Books, 2023.

Hyman, Mark. *Food: What the Heck Should I Eat?* New York, Little, Brown and Company, 2018.

Hyman, Mark. *Young Forever: The Secrets to Living Your Longest, Healthiest Life*. New York, Little, Brown and Company, 2023.

Fung, Jason. *The Obesity Code: Unlocking the Secrets of Weight Loss*. Vancouver, Greystone Books, 2016.

Fung, Jason. *The Diabetes Code: Prevent and Reverse Type 2 Diabetes Naturally*. Vancouver, Greystone Books, 2018.

Castillo, Brooke. *What's Possible*. [Publisher information not provided in search results], 2022.

Castillo, Brooke. *Stop Buffering: How to Manage Your Mind and Create the Life You Want*. [Publisher information not provided in search results], 2019.

McGraw, Phil. *The Ultimate Weight Solution: The 7 Keys to Weight Loss Freedom*. New York, Simon & Schuster, 2003.

McGraw, Phil. *Self Matters: Creating Your Life from the Inside Out*. New York, Threshold Editions, 2003.

Reno, Tosca. *Your Best Body Now: The 12-Week Plan to Turn Your Body into a Lean, Fat-Burning Machine*. Toronto, Harlequin, 2011.

Reno, Tosca. The Eat-Clean Diet: Recharged. New York, Hachette Books, 2010.

Michaels, Jillian. *The 6 Keys: Unlock Your Genetic Potential for Ageless Strength, Health, and Beauty*. New York, Hachette Books, 2018.

Michaels, Jillian. *Unlimited: How to Build an Exceptional Life*. New York, HarperCollins, 2009.

DiNicolantonio, James. The Obesity Fix: How to Beat Food Cravings, Lose Weight, and Gain Energy. Independently published, 2022.

DiNicolantonio, James, and Jason Fung. *The Longevity Solution: Rediscovering Centuries-Old Secrets to a Healthy, Long Life*. New York, HarperCollins, 2019.

Horton, Tony. Bring It!: How to Build Your Own Diet and Fitness Plan. New York, HarperCollins, 2008.

Horton, Tony. *The Big Picture: 11 Laws That Will Change Your Life*. New York, HarperCollins, 2014.

Freedom from Obesity

Michael Fatburner